Trace Elements in Renal Insufficiency

Contributions to Nephrology

Vol. 38

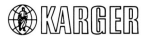

S. Karger · Basel · München · Paris · London · New York · Tokyo · Sydney

Trace Elements in Renal Insufficiency

Volume Editors
E.A. Quellhorst, Hann. Münden
K. Finke, Köln
C. Fuchs, Göttingen

54 figures and 30 tables, 1984

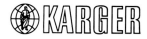

S. Karger · Basel · München · Paris · London · New York · Tokyo · Sydney

Contributions to Nephrology

National Library of Medicine, Cataloging in Publication
 Symposium on Trace Elements in Renal Insufficiency (1983: Bernried, Germany)
 Trace elements in renal insufficiency /
 Symposium on Trace Elements in Renal Insufficiency, Bernried, March 10–12, 1983.
 volume editors, E.A. Quellhorst, K. Finke, C. Fuchs. – Basel; New York: Karger, 1984.
 (Contributions to nephrology; v. 38)
 1. Kidney failure, chronic – metabolism – congresses 2. Trace elements – metabolism – congresses 3. Aluminum
 – metabolism – congresses 4. Metabolic diseases – etiology – congresses 5. Dialysis – congresses I. Quellhorst,
 E.A. (Eduard A.) II. Finke, K. (Klaus) III. Fuchs, Christoph IV. Title V. Series
 W1 CO778UN v. 38 [WJ 342 S989T 1983]
 ISBN 3-8055-3676-3

Drug Dosage
 The authors and the publisher have exerted every effort to ensure that drug selection and dosage set forth in this text
 are in accord with current recommendations and practice at the time of publication. However, in view of ongoing
 research, changes in government regulations, and the constant flow of information relating to drug therapy and drug
 reactions, the reader is urged to check the package insert for each drug for any change in indications and dosage and
 for added warnings and precautions. This is particularly important when the recommended agent is a new and/or
 infrequently employed drug.

Contents

Zinc Metabolism

Iron Metabolism

Magnesium Metabolism

Introduction

In patients with chronic renal insufficiency undergoing regular dialysis treatment the surface subjected to environmental influences is artificially enlarged by the dialyzer membrane area. Having been contaminated externally with incompatible substances via the membranes, the patients because of their restricted kidney function, are often not able to eliminate these by the natural pathways. Thus, many disturbances of our environment − for instance the increasing contamination with trace elements − being of little harm for healthy subjects may afflict dialysis patients in such a way as to induce severe metabolic derangements.

A symposium organized March 1983 in Bernried (Bavaria, FRG), sponsored by the German branch of Travenol, allowed for a profound and careful presentation and discussion on contemporary knowledge of trace element metabolism in renal insufficiency. Some new aspects concerning the metabolism of iron and magnesium seemed to justify the inclusion of these elements although they are not trace elements.

Undoubtedly, the loading of the organism with aluminium will increase rather than decrease in the near future. The increasing acidity of the soil, observed for almost one century (and not only as a consequence of contaminated moisture) will further augment the solubility of aluminium and thereby increase the aluminium content of tap water. Amongst other analytical problems, *R. Cornelis* points out the high aluminium content of the air which potentially contaminates samples before analysis and makes the results invalid. According to *J. Savory*, transfer of aluminium from the dialysis fluid into the patient's blood has to be anticipated unless the aluminium content of the dialysis fluid is extremely low (<10 µg/l). Another source of aluminium contamination, i.e. gastrointestinal absorption, is discussed by *O. Knoll*, who shows that high plasma aluminium levels can also be observed after aluminium hydroxide ingestion in patients even when using dialysis fluids with extremely low aluminium concentrations.

Dreams of the future are presented by *H. Schneider*, with his clinical observations after administration of an aluminium-free, atoxic natural polymer acting as an intestinal phosphate binder. The question whether serum aluminium concentrations reflect their tissue levels is raised by *M.E. De Broe* who shows that − at least as far as patients with osteomalacia are concerned − no correlation between serum and bone levels can be detected, with bone biopsy specimens giving the best available information about total body aluminium burden. In contradiction, *J.R. Winney* estimates the plasma aluminium as a sensitive index for the prevailing dialysis fluid aluminium concentration. According to his investigations, microcytic anaemia and osteomalacia are common signs of aluminium intoxication whereas encephalopathy occurs less frequently. The histological picture of aluminium osteopathy is described by *G.Cournot-Witmer* who suggests that aluminium present in the mitochondria of osteoblasts may intoxicate the cell thereby inducing the mineralization defect. Moreover, aluminium may have a direct toxic effect on the parathyroid glands, a fact which may explain low bone cell activity and turnover. According to *A. Pierides*, deferoxamine administration apart from kidney transplantation, is the treatment of choice in aluminium osteopathy, allowing the elimination of considerable amounts of aluminium during dialysis. A high binding capacity may prevent toxic reactions even if serum aluminium levels increase tremendously after deferoxamine administration (*P. Ackrill*). As referred to by *C. Fuchs* prophylactic measures such as the use of reverse osmosis for water preparation and the reduction of oral aluminium containing phosphate binders, do not guarantee he absence of aluminium intoxication; plasma aluminium determinations at intervals of 3 months are recommended.

Zinc metabolism in patients with chronic renal insufficiency is reviewed by *P.J. Aggett* who points out the difficulties in the determination of the nutritional status concerning this element, as plasma zinc levels represent only 0.5% of the total body zinc content. Restrictions of protein intake and administration of cation exchange resin or inorganic iron preparations may be responsible for zinc depletion in patients with chronic renal insufficiency. The question about zinc influencing sexual function in males remains undecided: Whereas *S.K. Mahajan* holds the 'Pro' position, demonstrating not only subjective influences on sexual function but also an increase of hormone levels during zinc supplementation, *R.S.C. Rodger* attempts to provide evidence via a double-blind study that this measure does not influence uraemic impotence. The position of *Rodger* is supported by *M. Schaefer* who observes no changes of hormonal parameters in spite of increasing plasma zinc levels during oral administration of this element and by *K.B.G. Sprenger*, who is not able to show an improvement of sexual dysfunction after zinc supplementation in the course of a double-blind study.

J.W. Eschbach summarizes iron kinetics in health and in renal insufficiency, identifying the important role of erythropoietin deficiency in renal impairment. Dialysis treatment may improve erythropoietic activity either by increased erythropoietin stimulation or, less probably, by elimination of inhibitors. According to *A. Blumberg*, patients on adequate dialysis treatment exhibit normal gastrointestinal iron absorption, with plasma ferritin measurements acting as reliable parameters for iron requirement. In children, the liver seems to represent body iron stores more reliably than bone marrow does (*D.E. Müller-Wiefel*). A disproportionate iron storage in the bone marrow and in the liver with a wide individual range is demonstrated by *F.L. van de Vyver* who uses laser techniques for the detection of iron in subcellular structures. Haemosiderosis as a consequence of iron overload or polytransfusion seems to exist in a small group of haemodialysis patients only and may be treated adequately by transplantation or deferoxamine (*Hilfenhaus*).

S.G. Massry refers to the distribution of magnesium in the various tissues of patients with chronic renal insufficiency, stressing that intestinal magnesium absorption in patients with renal insufficiency is no different from that of healthy individuals. The dangers of magnesium intoxication as a consequence of the ingestion of magnesium-containing antacids, especially in renal insufficiency, are represented by *C. Fuchs*. A survey on possibly existing interrelationships between magnesium metabolism and the development of renal osteodystrophy, given by *T. Drüeke*, concludes the symposium. The chairmen of the different sections were bothered with summaries of the discussions, a task, for which the editors have to express their deep gratitude.

Until a few years ago, the attention of all those responsible for the treatment of patients with renal insufficiency was directed towards the maintenance of their physical existence. Meanwhile, improvement of medical care and technical progress have succeeded in prolonging the life expectancy in this increasing group of patients. The occurrence of severe clinically evident derangements has been replaced by the appearance of disorders remaining almost undetected. In this respect, disturbances of trace element metabolism deserve our special consideration.

E. Quellhorst

Aluminium Metabolism

Contr. Nephrol., vol. 38, pp. 1–11 (Karger, Basel 1984)

Analytical Problems Related to Al-Determination in Body Fluids, Water and Dialysate

Rita Cornelis[1], Patrick Schutyser

Laboratory for Analytical Chemistry, Institute for Nuclear Sciences, University of Ghent, Belgium

Introduction

Any effort to reduce the health hazard caused by aluminum in patients with renal insufficiency brings analytical chemistry to the foreground. The latter is expected to ensure accurate and precise analytical data for Al in the various body fluids, in water and dialysate. The time has now come to assess certain methods and to improve the expertise. Both these requirements clearly impose themselves in the light of a selection of data published since 1974 on Al in plasma or serum, as well as in blood and urine of normal, healthy individuals. Table I groups 19 mean values of Al in serum or plasma. They cover the range between 2.1 and 42 µg Al $\cdot$ l^{-1}: 17 results were obtained by graphite furnace atomic absorption spectrometry, one by inductively coupled plasma atomic emission spectrometry and one by neutron activation analysis. Normal blood mean Al concentrations, also presented in table I, extend from 1.6 to 211 µg $\cdot$ l^{-1}. Mean Al urine levels, as given in table I, vary between 4.7 and 1,700 µg $\cdot$ l^{-1}. The question arises as to which data represents the true Al contents of normal serum, blood or urine, and whether the differences found should be ascribed to analytical errors rather than to biological variation.

---

[1] Senior Research Associate, National Fund for Scientific Research.

Table I. Normal Al concentrations in serum or plasma, blood and urine

Authors	Analytical technique	Mean μg · l⁻¹	SD μg · l⁻¹	Range μg · l⁻¹	Subjects n
Serum or plasma					
Alderman and Gitelman, 1980 [1]	AAS	2.1	2.2	0.0−7.6	14
Oster, 1981 [2]	AAS	<4		<2.5−7	37
Leung and Henderson, 1982 [3]	AAS	6.5	4.1	2−14	28
Kaehny et al., 1977 [4]	AAS	7	2		13
Parkinson et al., 1982 [5]	AAS	7.3		2−15	46
Gardiner et al., 1981 [6]	AAS	10.2		3.2−32.4	15
Salvadeo et al., 1979 [7]	AAS	12.0	4.0		12
Wawschinek et al., 1982 [8]	AAS	14.0ᵃ		3.0−39.0	54
Gilli et al., 1980 [9]	AAS	14.15	12.2		44
Valentin et al., 1976 [10]	AAS	14ᵃ	7.1	4.0−34.5	40
Elliott et al., 1978 [11]	AAS	16.2			20
Zumkley et al., 1979 [12]	AAS	23.20	7.29		20
Clavel et al., 1978 [13]	AAS	24	8	10−45	59
Ward et al., 1978 [14]	NAA	25		10−50	10
Gorsky and Dietz, 1978 [15]	AAS	28	9	12−46	23
Pegon, 1978 [16]	AAS	34.1	3.5	28−40	20
McKinney et al., 1982 [17]	AAS	35	3.7		7
Fuchs et al., 1974 [18]	AAS	38ᶜ		10−92	29
Schramel and Wolf, 1980 [19]	ICP-AES	42	16	20−75	20
Blood					
Frech et al., 1982 [20]	AAS	1.6ᵇ	1.29		11
		7.5	6.41		43
Allain and Mauras, 1979 [21]	ICP-AES	12.5	4.0		14
Langmyhr and Tsalev, 1977 [22]	AAS	211ᶜ		53−622	48
Urine					
Allain und Mauras, 1979 [21]	ICP-AES	4.7	2.5		14
Leung and Henderson, 1982 [3]	AAS	<10			
Kaehny et al., 1977 [4]	AAS	13	5		13
Valentin et al., 1976 [10]	AAS	17ᵃ		3.5−31.0	32
Gorsky and Dietz, 1978 [15]	AAS	45ᵈ	32	6−92	12
Blotcky et al., 1976 [23]	NAA			<50−130	6
Lichte et al., 1980 [24]	ICP-AES			200−1,700	4

AAS = Atomic absorption spectrometry; ICP-AES = inductively coupled plasma atomic emission spectrometry; NAA = neutron activation analysis.
ᵃMedian; ᵇclass-100 atmosphere; values not corrected for blank; ᶜrecalculated values; assuming a serum- or blood-specific density of 1.026 or 1.055, respectively; ᵈdaily excretion.

Sample Collecting and Handling Procedures

A first prerequisite consists in keeping the biological sample, water or dialysate unaltered in terms of Al content throughout the sampling steps. Contamination through Al is one of the major factors invalidating Al analyses at the microgram per liter level and appears to be a greater hazard than the opposite, namely losses. Errors due to extraneous additions are very difficult to estimate. They are random in nature and come out of the air, vessels, chemicals, the analyst himself.

A major source of Al is airborne. Table II gives an idea of the Al content of dust deposits, as measured in our laboratory. There is a remarkable 9-fold decrease in the Al content in a clean-air laboratory as compared to a usual analytical environment. This is not surprising as Al is one of the most abundant elements in the earth crust and constitutes about 1.5% of the dust in the household.

Al is also a common constituent of laboratory ware and ultrapure acids. Data for glass, polyethylene (low pressure and high pressure), polypropylene and for hydrochloric, hydrofluoric and nitric acids can be read in table II. Extended storage of the ultrapure acids can increase the concentration by a factor up to 10. Al can also be leached out of the containers by e.g. acids (table II) [26].

From the above description there follows that exploration of microgram per liter contents of Al requires the following precautions: (1) clean room conditions (fall-out $< 1 \, \mu g \, Al \cdot m^{-2} \cdot day^{-1}$); (2) high-purity collecting and storage vessels, rigorously cleaned and leached with ultrapure acids and water, some authors advise EDTA solutions [3, 27, 39]; (3) contamination-free sampling and handling of blood (no anticoagulant), urine, dialysate and water; (4) correct choice of analytical technique, with regards to both as to sensitivity and accuracy.

The reward of all these painstaking efforts is reflected in a recent publication by *Frech* et al. [20]. They reported a mean Al value in whole blood of $7.5 \pm 6.11 \, \mu g \, Al \cdot l^{-1}$ in 43 normal individuals (table I). The values were corrected for a blank of $1.0 \pm 0.59 \, \mu g \cdot l^{-1}$. These samples were taken and processed in hospital surroundings, taking the usual analytical precautions. They repeated their experiments with blood samples from 11 different healthy volunteers, sampled and handled in a controlled class 100 atmosphere. They then obtained a mean Al value of $1.6 \pm 1.29 \, \mu g \, Al \cdot l^{-1}$ (values not corrected for blank). This data did not fit well into a normal distribution. A statistical evaluation revealed, however, that the true mean value of the

Table II. Sources of Al contamination: air fall-out, laboratory ware, ultrapure acids and amounts leached out by HCl and HNO_3 from plastics [25]

	Al content
Air fall-out	
Outdoors	$179 \, \mu g \cdot m^{-2} \cdot day^{-1}$
Analytical laboratory	$8.2 \, \mu g \cdot m^{-2} \cdot day^{-1}$
Clean-air laboratory	$0.9 \, \mu g \cdot m^{-2} \cdot day^{-1}$
Laboratory ware	
Glass	$100 \, \mu g \cdot g^{-1}$
Polyethylene (LP)	$100 \, \mu g \cdot g^{-1}$
Teflon	$0.1-10 \, \mu g \cdot g^{-1}$
Polyethylene (HP)	$0.01-0.1 \, \mu g \cdot g^{-1}$
Polypropylene	$0.01-0.1 \, \mu g \cdot g^{-1}$
Ultrapure acids	
HCl	$1 \, \mu g \cdot l^{-1}$
HF	$0.1-1 \, \mu g \cdot l^{-1}$
HNO_3	$0.1-1 \, \mu g \cdot l^{-1}$

	Al leached out after 1 week's contact $ng \cdot cm^{-2}$	
	$6N$ HCl	$9N$ HNO_3
Material		
Polyethylene (HP)	10	
Polyethylene (LP)	$1-10$	
Polycarbonate	$1-10$	$1-10$
Teflon	$1-10$	$1-10$

HP = High pressure; LP = low pressure.

blood samples is, with 96.5% probability, higher than the true mean value of the blank. In other words, the normal Al blood or serum content often lies below the current level of detection and hence is not quantifiable.

Another factor which endangers the integrity of the sample is loss of Al from the solution through adsorption on the container wall. This is dependant on the chemical composition of the sample (acidity, stability, concentration, chemical form) and on the nature of the collection vial (material, surface). Experimental evidence has shown that $< 100\,\mu g\;Al \cdot l^{-1}$ water makes the analysis within 24 h essential. Acidification can, however, prevent losses due to adsorption. Some researchers advise freezing at $-20\,°C$ [28]. As far as storage of serum samples is concerned, it seems that refrigeration at $4 - 10\,°C$ is preferable to deep freezing, which may denature serum proteins, leading to inhomogeneous samples [29, 39].

Analytical Requirements

Analytical requirements for Al determination differ according to the objective pursued and the matrix studied. First of all comes serum or plasma, with three distinct concentration ranges of particular interest: (1) normal serum: $<10\,\mu g\;Al \cdot l^{-1}$, if not $<1\,\mu g\;Al \cdot l^{-1}$: these determinations are only accessible to a few laboratories, since a sensitivity of $0.1\,\mu g\;Al \cdot l^{-1}$ is indispensable; (2) patients with renal insufficiency moderately exposed to Al: $50-200\,\mu g\;Al \cdot l^{-1}$ serum; (3) patients exposed to Al showing clinical signs of intoxication: $300-1,000\,\mu g\;Al \cdot l^{-1}$ serum. Every clinical laboratory equipped for these Al analyses should be able to deal with the last two groups, as with the matrix effects not only of the serum but also those caused by urine, dialysate or unpurified domestic water. For Al determinations in pure water or dialysate, a sensitivity of $1\,\mu g\;Al \cdot l^{-1}$ is recommended.

Methods

This paragraph only bears on those analytical techniques which make it possible to handle the large number of samples one faces in clinical practice. One or the other of two types of spectrometry can be used: (1) atomic absorption spectrometry (AAS), more specifically graphite furnace atomic absorption spectrometry (GFAAS); (2) atomic emission spectrometry (AES), more particularly inductively coupled plasma AES (ICP-AES). For information on both theory and practical application of AAS the books by *Ebdon* [30] and *Kirkbright and Sargent* [31] should be consulted, on ICP-AES the publications by *Fassel and Kniseley* [32], *Robin* [33] and *Boumans and Lux-Steiner* [34]. Photometric determinations of Al will only be dealt with briefly. Up to a decade ago, they were extensively studied [35], but they are now losing field in favor of AAS and ICP-AES.

Graphite Furnace Atomic Absorption Spectrometry

GFAAS still holds the greatest potentialities and is the method of choice in the dialysis centers currently screening serum, dialysate and water Al contents. The atomic absorbance of Al is normally monitored at 309.3 nm, with a spectral band width of 0.7 nm. The furnace is purged with Ar during the operation. The temperature program consists of drying, charring, ashing and atomization steps and must be optimized according to each laboratory's instrumentation and sample pretreatment procedures.

In the case of serum, the simplest pretreatment is 4- to 6-fold dilution with water [6]. Centrifugation on the diluted sample is advisable to remove debris prior to the autosampler injection of e.g. 20 µl into the oven. This simple dilution technique also reduces matrix effects and carbon buildup. Some researchers dilute with Triton X-100 or perform a complete mineralization of serum or blood. The latter procedure is, however, time-consuming and much more prone to contamination. Dialysate is also preferably diluted.

GFAAS is subject to various physical and chemical interferences and to background absorption, the nature and extent of which may vary in the different kinds of atomizers [30]. Physical interferences can be expected because of the steep thermal gradient in the graphite tube. As a consequence any variation in the sample position (e.g. because of pipetting, surface tension or viscosity) alters the atomization peak. A rapid heating ramp and an isothermal operation will help to minimize the problem. A small graphite L'vov platform inside the tube on which the sample is deposited already solves some of the difficulties. The platform is essentially heated by radiation from the tube walls. Consequently, its heating is delayed and both vaporization and atomization will take place in an environment of relatively high and constant temperature and thus be more favorable to the dissociation of the molecules [3, 20].

Chemical interferences may be very frustrating when measuring Al in serum, blood, urine or dialysate. Al is expected to volatilize to Al oxide species prior to atomization at a temperature of about 2,700°C, but residual compounds containing H, O, N, Cl or S affect this process [36]. As the samples to be analyzed are rich in e.g. Cl^-, some volatile Al chlorides could be produced, which have a high dissociation energy and lead to loss by lack of atomization. Therefore the use of HCl in GFAAS Al detection is to be avoided. Some authors report stabilization procedures often referred to as matrix modification. This not only reduces losses on ashing, but also permits the use of higher ashing temperatures. This tends to minimize background and other matrix effects. Modifiers used are $Mg(NO_3)_2$ [3], ammonium EDTA or EDTA and $NH_4(OH)$ [39]. Moreover, anion and cation interferences can occur and bring about a decrease in the absorption signal. These interferences are usually remedied by matching standards and samples (a most difficult task) or by the method of standard additions.

Another chemical interference may be due to the graphite tube, which is porous and exhibits a tendency toward carbide formation. The surface of the tube also changes in composition after repeated firing cycles and this in turn affects the atomization efficiency. These disadvantages are inevitable with Al, but can be partially overcome by the use of pyrolytic tubes (obtained by heating the tubes in a methane atmosphere), which are far less porous.

Except in the case of Al determination in very pure water, automatic, simultaneous background correction is practically essential, as nonspecific absorption in the furnace is very severe. Molecules may exhibit absorption spectra in the specific 309.3 nm region of Al. Smoke from the organic substances of serum, blood or urine further complicates the matter. Light emission from the incandescent walls may further distort the baseline. The classic deuterium background correction deals with all this, the recently introduced Zeeman effect AAS even better [37].

The readout can be either peak height of the transient absorption signal or peak area measurement, which is more precise. A display of graphical recording of the net absorption signal and its background is a most useful diagnostic tool for the analyst. The overall precision of Al determination by GFAAS is between 3 and 10% and is poorest near the detection limit (5, 1, 0.1 µg Al · l^{-1} depending on the equipment).

Inductively Coupled Plasma Atomic Emission Spectrometry

This method is more elaborate and entails more expense than GFAAS, but has the advantage of being a multielement technique featuring a comparable sensitivity to GFAAS for many elements. The excitation source is an inductively coupled Ar plasma which can attain temperatures of 6,000−7,000 K, which explains the much improved detection limits in comparison with flame or arc AES. The detection limit for Al is reported to be 1 µg · l^{-1} [38], but is more likely to be 5−10 times higher when resorting to commerical equipment. The calibration curve is linear over three to five orders of magnitude. This can be explained by the absence of self-absorption up to high Al concentrations.

Although physical and chemical interferences do occur, the matrix effects can be sufficiently controlled or suppressed to yield accurate results [33]. The liquid sample has first of all to be *nebulized*. This process is influenced by the sample's viscosity and surface tension. Both parameters are important in case of serum, blood or urine due to their contents in organic substances and salts. Dialysate also exhibits this major drawback of salt effect during nebulization. This kind of interference can be avoided by choosing an adequate nebulizer and by matching standard and sample solutions.

Volatilization interference is caused by occlusion of Al in matrix particles created during the transport of the sample aerosol to the plasma. Consequently the volatilization behavior of plasma Al is predominantly governed by the matrix characteristics.

Atomization of the sample is also subject to interference by the matrix components. Calcium, e.g., forms a compound with Al which is difficult to dissociate. This can result in an incomplete atomization of the Al-containing compound, and, hence, in the signal suppression for Al. Volatilization and atomization interferences can be greatly reduced by increasing the power input in the Ar plasma.

The next process to consider is the *ionization* of the analyte atoms. An important plasma characteristic is the electron number density, which influences the atom-ion equilibrium and, hence, the intensities of the respective atom and ion lines. Remarkably enough, the introduction in the Ar plasma of samples containing high alkali-metal concentrations does not significantly increase the electron number density in the plasma. It is not yet fully understood why ICP-AES is relatively insensitive to this ionization interference. This limited influence can be totally avoided by careful selection of the experimental conditions.

Finally, spectrometric interference can occur during *excitation*. When Al is measured at 394.40 nm in the presence of Ca, the broad emission line of Ca at 393.37 nm causes an important spectral background shift at the analytical wavelength considered. This interference can be handled by applying background correction techniques and appropriate computation.

The stability of the plasma excitation source is particularly good: 0.1−0.3% a day. When actual measurements are carried out with aqueous solutions, the precision deteriorates to approximately 2−3%, depending upon the nebulizer and spray chamber chosen.

Photometry

UV-visible spectrophotometric determinations of Al are based on the measurement of molecular complexes of Al, either by colorimetry or fluorimetry [35]. These procedures are still currently used for the determination of low concentrations of dissolved Al in water [28] and dialysate. However, they are subject to many interferences by other ions or by organic material. Photometry is not the method of choice for Al determinations in serum, blood or urine as this would involve very time-consuming matrix destructions and adequate interference studies.

Reliability of Analytical Data

Trace element investigations are only significant if supported by accurate and precise analytical data. Precision is synonymous with repeatability, whereas accuracy points out the 'true' content. An invaluable asset for a laboratory trying to detect its own errors is the availability of standard reference materials (SRMs), with a matrix similar to the sample studied and certified for trace and ultratrace element content.

There existed a water SRM 1643 issued by the National Bureau of Standards, Washington with a certified content of 77 ± 1 ng Al $\cdot$ g^{-1} H$_2$O. Unfortunately this SRM is exhausted and has been replaced by the water SRM 1643−a, lacking certification for Al. In the meantime the US Environmental Protection Agency has provided a water quality control sample with known Al content, which is available on request (Environmental Protection Agency, Quality Assurance Branch, Environmental Monitoring and Support Laboratory, US EPA, Cincinnati, OH 45268).

Biological SRMs with certified Al content are inexistent. Any laboratory investigating microgram Al $\cdot$ l^{-1} levels is, however, in need of strict quality control and, to that end, serum, dialysate and water SRMs certified for Al are basic necessities. SRMs do not as yet exist, though they remain vital for a better understanding of the intrinsic role of Al in the human body.

References

1   Alderman, F.; Gitelman, H.: Improved electrothermal determination of aluminum in serum by atomic absorption spectroscopy. Clin. Chem. *26*: 258−260 (1980).
2   Oster, O.: The aluminium content of human serum determined by atomic absorption spectroscopy with a graphite furnace. Clinica chim. Acta *114*: 53−60 (1981).

3 Leung, F.; Henderson, A.: Improved determination of aluminum in serum and urine with use of a stabilized temperature platform furnace. Clin. Chem. *28*: 2139–2143 (1982).

4 Kaehny, W.; Alfrey, A.; Holman, R.; Schorr, W.: Aluminum transfer during hemodialysis. Kidney int. *12*: 361–365 (1977).

5 Parkinson, I.; Ward, M.; Kerr, D.: A method for the routine determination of aluminium in serum and water by flameless atomic absorption spectrometry. Clinica chim. Acta *125*: 125–133 (1982).

6 Gardiner, P.; Ottaway, J.; Fell, G.; Halls, D.: Determination of aluminium in blood plasma or serum by electrothermal atomic absorption spectrometry. Analytica chim. Acta *128*: 57–66 (1981).

7 Salvadeo, A.; Minoia, C.; Segagni, S.; Villa, G.: Trace metal changes in dialysis fluid and blood of patients on hemodialysis. Int. J. artif. Organs *2*: 17–21 (1979).

8 Wawschinek, O.; Petek, W.; Lang, J.; Pogglitsch, H.; Holzer, H.: The determination of aluminium in human plasma. Mikrochim. Acta *1*: 335–339 (1982).

9 Gilli, P.; Farinelli, A.; Fagioli, F.; De Bastiani, P.; Buoncristiani, U.: Serum aluminium levels in patients on peritoneal dialysis. Lancet *ii*: 742–743 (1980).

10 Valentin, H.; Preusser, P.; Schaller, K.: Die Analyse von Aluminium in Serum und Urin zur Überwachung exponierter Personen. Int. Archs. occup. environ. Hlth *38*: 1–17 (1976).

11 Elliott, H.; Dryburgh, F.; Fell, G.; Sabet, S.; MacDougall, A.: Aluminium toxicity during regular hemodialysis. Br. med. J. *i*: 1101–1103 (1978).

12 Zumkley, H.; Bertram, H.; Lison, A.; Knoll, O.; Losse, H.: Aluminium, zinc and copper concentrations in plasma in chronic renal insufficiency. Clin. Nephrol. *12*: 18–21 (1979).

13 Clavel, J.; Jaudon, M.; Galli, A.: Dosage de l'aluminium dans les liquides biologiques par spectrophotométrie d'absorption atomique en four graphite. Annls. Biol. clin. *36*: 33–38 (1978).

14 Ward, M.; Feest, T.; Ellis, H.; Parkinson, I.; Kerr, D.: Osteomalacic dialysis osteodystrophy: evidence for a water-borne aetiological agent, probably aluminium. Lancet *i*: 841–845 (1978).

15 Gorsky, J.; Dietz, A.: Determination of aluminum in biological samples by atomic absorption spectrophotometry with a graphite furnace. Clin. Chem. *24*: 1485–1490 (1978).

16 Pegon, Y.: Dosage de l'aluminium dans les liquides biologiques par absorption atomique sans flamme. Analytica chim. Acta *101*: 385–391 (1978).

17 McKinney, T.; Basinger, M.; Dawson, E.; Jones, M.: Serum aluminum levels in dialysis dementia. Nephron *32*: 53–56 (1982).

18 Fuchs, C.; Brasche, M.; Paschen, K.; Nordbeck, H.; Quellhorst, E.: Aluminium-Bestimmung im Serum mit flammenloser Atomabsorption. Clinica chim. Acta *52*: 71–80 (1974).

19 Schramel, P.; Wolf, A.: Direktbestimmung von Aluminium in Serumproben mittels inductively coupled Plasma-Emissionsspektralanalyse. J. clin. Chem. clin. Biochem. *18*: 591–593 (1980).

20 Frech, W.; Cedergren, A.; Cederberg, C.; Vessman, J.: Evaluation of some critical factors affecting determination of aluminum in blood, plasma or serum by electrothermal atomic absorption spectroscopy. Clin. Chem. *28*: 2259–2263 (1982).

21   Allain, P.; Mauras, Y.: Determination of aluminum in blood, urine and water by induc-
      tively coupled plasma emission spectrometry. Analyt. Chem. 51: 2089−2091 (1979).

22   Langmyhr, F.; Tsalev, D.: Atomic absorption spectrometric determination of
      aluminium in whole blood. Analytica chim. Acta 92: 79−83 (1977).

23   Blotcky, A.; Hobson, D.; Leffler, J.; Rack, E.; Recker, R.: Determination of trace
      aluminum in urine by neutron activation analysis. Analyt. Chem. 48: 1084−1088 (1976).

24   Lichte, F.; Hopper, S.; Osborn, T.: Determination of silicon and aluminum in biological
      matrices by inductively coupled plasma emission spectrometry. Analyt. Chem. 52:
      120−124 (1980).

25   Kosta, L.: Contamination as a limiting parameter in trace analysis. Talanta 29: 985−992
      (1982).

26   Moody, J.; Lindstrom, R.: Selection and cleaning of platic containers for storage of
      trace element samples. Analyt. Chem. 49: 2264−2267 (1977).

27   Smeyers-Verbeke, J.; Verbeelen, D.; Massart, D.: The determination of aluminum in
      biological fluids by means of graphite furnace atomic absorption spectrometry. Clinica
      chim. Acta 108: 67−73 (1980).

28   Hydes, D.; Liss, P.: Fluorimetric method for the determination of low concentrations
      of dissolved aluminum in natural waters. Analyst 101: 922−931 (1976).

29   Bertram, H.: Aluminiumbestimmung in Körperflüssigkeiten. Nieren-Hochdruck-
      krankh. 10: 188−191 (1981).

30   Ebdon, L.: An introduction to atomic absorption spectroscopy (Heyden & Son, London
      1982).

31   Kirkbright, F.; Sargent, M.: Atomic absorption and fluorescence spectroscopy
      (Academic Press, London 1974).

32   Fassel, V.; Kniseley, R.: Inductively coupled plasma-optical emission spectroscopy.
      Analyt. Chem. 46: 1110A−1120A (1974).

33   Robin, J.: Emission spectrometry with the aid of an inductive plasma generator. ICP
      Inf. Newsl. 4: 495−509 (1979).

34   Boumans, P.; Lux-Steiner, M.: Modification and optimization of a 50 MHz inductively
      coupled argon plasma with special reference to analyses using organic solvents. Spec-
      trochim. Acta 37B: 97−126 (1982).

35   Fresenius, W.; Jander, G.: Handbuch der analytischen Chemie. Elemente der dritten
      Hauptgruppe, pp. 275−469 (Springer, Berlin 1972).

36   Persson, J.; Frech, W.; Cedergren, A.: Investigations of reactions involved in flameless
      atomic absorption procedures. Part. IV. A theoretical study of factors influencing the
      determination of Al. Analytica chim. Acta 92: 85−93 (1977).

37   Brown, S.: Zeeman effect-based background correction in atomic absorption spec-
      trometry. Analyt. Chem. 49: 1269A−1281A (1977).

38   Boumans, P.; Barnes, R.: Detection limits 1978. ICP Inf. Newsl. 3: 445−448 (1978).

39   Fell, G.: Electrothermal atomic spectrophotometric analysis of Al in blood serum or
      plasma. Ann. clin. Lab. Sci. (in press, 1983).

Dr. Rita Cornelis, Laboratory for Analytical Chemistry, Institute for Nuclear Sciences,
Rijksuniversiteit Gent, Proeftuinstraat 86, B-9000 Gent (Belgium)

Contr. Nephrol., vol. 38, pp. 12–23 (Karger, Basel 1984)

Dialysis Fluids as a Source of Aluminum Accumulation

John Savory, Michael R. Wills

Departments of Pathology, Biochemistry, and Internal Medicine, University of Virginia Medical Center, Charlottesville, Va., USA

A number of clinical disorders in patients with chronic renal failure on long-term intermittent hemodialysis have been related to aluminum toxicity [1, 2, 6, 7, 21]. The two potential sources for the increased tissue aluminum content are transfer across the dialysis membrane from aluminum in the water used in the preparation of the dialysate and intestinal absorption from aluminum-containing phosphate-binding gels [15, 18, 21, 23]. Knowledge of the uptake of aluminum, particularly from the dialysate, is of considerable importance in understanding disorders related to aluminum toxicity. In addition, the binding of aluminum to various constituents of blood, especially in the extracellular compartment, must play an important role in the transport of aluminum to target tissues.

This present review surveys the limited information on the distribution of aluminum species in the plasma of normals and hemodialysis patients and also the transfer of aluminum during hemodialysis.

Following the uptake of aluminum from either the dialysate or after oral ingestion, between 50 and 70% is in the plasma, and the remainder is associated mainly with erythrocytes; very little information is available on aluminum distribution in whole blood.

Distribution in Plasma

Kaehny et al. [14] studied aluminum transfer during hemodialysis from a dialysate with a low aluminum concentration to blood with an elevated concentration. Aluminum appeared to be strongly bound to a serum or plasma component, but the binding sites apparently were saturable, since plasma aluminum values reach a plateau during the dialysis procedure.

Table I. Ultrafiltrable aluminum in normals subjects

n	Aluminum concentration µg/l		Protein binding, %
	serum	ultrafiltrate	
10	40.2 ± 7.2	18.2 ± 1.8	59.0 ± 5.8

Using ultrafiltration techniques, several investigators have reported protein-bound and nonprotein-bound fractions of plasma aluminum. *Lundin* et al. [19] studied the partition of aluminum in the plasma of 10 normal individuals using ultrafiltration with membranes having a cutoff of 6,000–8,000 daltons. The results obtained are shown in table I; the protein binding averaged 59% of total serum aluminum.

Elliott et al. [6] in a brief communication reported that more than 70% of the aluminum in blood was present in the plasma compartment. In normal subjects, they reported that a very small proportion of the plasma aluminum was ultrafiltrable. These findings were not consistent with those of *Lundin* et al. [19]. In the study of *Elliott* et al. [6] the tendency was for the ultrafiltrable fraction to decrease as the total plasma aluminum concentration fell below 200 µg/l. At higher plasma aluminum levels, studies using polyethylene glycol and direct ultrafiltration indicated that 60–70% of the aluminum was bound to high-molecular weight proteins, 10–20% was bound to albumin, and 10–30% was ultrafiltrable.

Graf et al. [10, 11] performed in vivo ultrafiltration studies on patients during hemodialysis. Their results revealed an ultrafiltration fraction of about 20% of total plasma aluminum, suggesting that 80% of the aluminum was protein bound.

It is apparent that more detailed information is needed of aluminum distribution in the plasma of normals and patients on chronic intermittent hemodialysis. Such information would clarify the variability of reports on aluminum loading during hemodialysis. Recent work in the authors' laboratory [16, 17] has been directed towards an attempt to separate aluminum species in plasma into more than just ultrafiltrable and protein-bound fractions. The approach used to define the plasma distribution and binding of aluminum was to employ gel filtration under equilibrium conditions which was a technique used previously in our laboratory for studying the distribution of calcium in plasma [25].

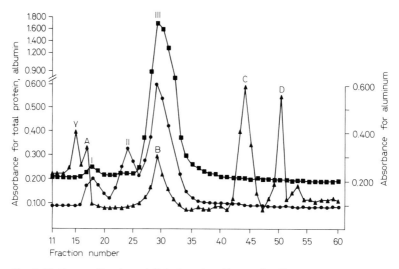

Fig. 1. Elution profile of renal dialysis patient [from ref. 16]. ● = Total protein; ■ = albumin; ▲ = aluminum. For explanation of other symbols see text.

Separations were carried out on a column packed with Sephacryl S-200 superfine with a column eluent containing per liter 140 mmol Na^+, 1.1 mmol Ca^{++}, 0.5 mmol Mg^{++}, 4.0 mmol K^+, and 10 mmol 2-[tris(hydroxy-methyl)-methyl]aminoethanesulfonic acid (TES) adjusted to pH 7.40 at 37°C. This eluting solution was analyzed, and the aluminum concentration was found to be 11 µg/l.

The typical elution profile for a patient on renal dialysis (fig. 1) was similar to the pattern obtained in a normal subject [17]. The first aluminum peak (Y) which eluted before peak A was not present in the serum from the normal volunteer [17].

The aluminum in the peak Y which created a species large enough to be excluded from the column must be complexed in some manner. Such a complex might be with protein, lipoprotein, cholesterol, or triglycerides. The fractions containing the aluminum in this peak were analyzed for cholesterol and triglyceride in order to determine if any lipid material containing these compounds was present, but none was detected. However, this observation could have been due to the relatively low sensitivity of the methods used. Since aluminum is capable of forming colloids, the aluminum may have been complexed in a colloidal species which would be excluded from the column and thus elute in the void volume. Neither the composition of the aluminum nor the significance of the aluminum in peak Y is understood. However, this peak has been present in the elution profile of 4 renal patients and has not been seen in the profile using serum from a normal volunteer.

Aluminum in peak A was associated with some high molecular weight proteins present in the early elution of protein peak 1. This peak has been previously shown to contain alpha-2-macroglobulin, IgM, haptoglobin, and some orosomucoid [25]. The present study has not provided information as to whether all of these proteins, a single one, or an undetected protein provides the binding of aluminum.

The aluminum in peak B was eluted in association with the albumin in peak III, and this amount of aluminum was greater in dialysis patients than in a normal volunteer [17], undoubtedly due to the higher aluminum concentration in the serum of the dialysis patients. The two largest aluminum peaks were peaks C and D. The nature of these peaks was studied by repeating the gel filtration procedure using a free eluent potassium and monitoring the eluted protein with an UV detector. The column fractions were analyzed for potassium and aluminum, and the results are shown in figure 2. The elution pattern was similar to that seen in figure 1. The greater separation between the aluminum peaks C and D in figures 1 and 2 was due to the slower flow rate used in the latter run.

The aluminum in peak C was probably bound to small inorganic species, such as phosphate and bicarbonate, which were reported to elute just before the potassium peak in a calcium-binding study using the same gel filtration technique employed here [25]. However, the aluminum also might have been associated with the protein material in this peak, as shown by absorbance at 280 nm. The aluminum in peak D was associated with a group of proteins and/or small polypeptides, as indicated by peak IV. Using polyacrylamide gel electrophoresis, two proteins were found under this peak with apparent molecular weights of 60,000 and 80,000. These proteins must have appeared in the later column fractions because of retardation owing to some interaction with the Sephacryl S-200 gel. Since amylase is known to interact with these type gels, the fractions were analyzed for amylase activity, and none was found. At this time the identities of these two proteins are not known.

In order to investigate the effect of exposing plasma to aluminum and imitating hemodialysis with aluminum-contaminated dialysate, the serum from the renal patient used in figure 1 was chromatographed with an eluting buffer containing approximately 90 µg/l of aluminum. In this procedure,

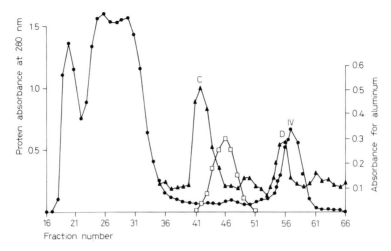

Fig. 2. Elution profile with potassium-free buffer and ultraviolet detector [from ref. 16].
● = Protein; ▲ = aluminum; □ = potassium. For explanation of other symbols see text.

the serum constituents that bind aluminum would take up aluminum from
the buffer and possibly mimic the plasma binding of the aluminum that
crosses the dialysis membrane. The elution pattern obtained with the added
aluminum revealed an increase in the aluminum in peak A and caused
peaks C and D to become one broad peak. No increase in the amount of
aluminum bound to albumin or the peak in the void volume (peak Y) was
observed. These results are consistent with the view that albumin is easily
saturated with aluminum, and the excess aluminum must be bound to other
serum constituents.

Transfer during Hemodialysis

The transfer of aluminum from the dialysate across the dialysis membrane into the patient's bloodstream during hemodialysis appears to occur
even when the dialysate aluminum concentration is low [14]. *Kaehny* et al.
[14] reported on a study of patients from a unit (A) which had a low
aluminum dialysate concentration and from a second unit (B-1) with a high
aluminum dialysate concentration. The study was repeated in some of the
patients from unit B after the aluminum content of the dialysate was re-

Table II. Plasma aluminum during hemodialysis

| Unit | n | Plasma aluminum concentration µg/l | |
		beforedialysis	afterdialysis
A	14	55 ± 28	59 ± 26
B-1	18	162 ± 66	303 ± 76
B-2	14	84 ± 28	114 ± 39

Table III. Plasma aluminum during hemodialysis

| n | Plasma aluminum concentrations µg/l | |
	beforedialysis	afterdialysis
45	93 ± 29	99 ± 35

duced (study B-2). The results are shown in table II. There were significant increases in plasma aluminum during hemodialysis. These workers also demonstrated that the urine excretion of aluminum in a group of patients dialyzed against a dialysate with a high aluminum concentration was greater than that in patients dialyzed against a low-aluminum dialysate. These findings are consistent with the view that aluminum loading occurs during dialysis. A similar study was carried out in the authors' laboratory [16] using a dialysate with a low (7 µg/l) aluminum concentration. The results are shown in table III and showed a statistically significant increase in the serum aluminum concentrations of these patients following the hemodialysis procedure (t test, $p < 0.001$). Both studies showed increased serum aluminum concentrations after dialysis, even when the dialysate aluminum concentration was as low as 5 µg/l in the study of *Kaehny* et al. [14] and 7 µg/l in the authors' investigation. From these studies one can conclude that some aluminum can be transferred to plasma during dialysis, if the dialysate contains virtually no aluminum. The inference is that aluminum is tightly bound to one of the nondialyzable plasma constituents discussed earlier. This binding also makes it extremely difficult to remove the aluminum from the patient during dialysis.

Kovalchik et al. [18] studied the transfer of aluminum across the dialysis membrane in dogs during hemodialysis and monitored the simultaneous urinary and biliary excretion of aluminum. Their study was carried out in two groups of dogs: in one group the ureters were ligated, while in the second group the ureters were left intact. Blood samples were taken in each group at 30 and 60 min prior to the start of hemodialysis, and the aluminum concentration in these samples was used as the control. Plasma aluminum values increased in both groups of dogs during a 4-hour dialysis period. During the postdialysis period, the plasma aluminum values in the ligated group remained elevated, while the values in the normal group returned to a concentration that was not significantly different from the control values. The urine excretion of aluminum also increased during dialysis and then decreased during the postdialysis period in the nonligated dogs. The dogs excreted 37% of the total aluminum load during the dialysis and the postdialysis periods. The findings in that study are consistent with the theory that aluminum is bound in the plasma compartment, since the peak plasma values were greater than that of the dialysate, and less than half of the plasma aluminium was excreted.

In contrast, however, to the findings of *Kovalchik* et al. [18], who showed that aluminum concentration in plasma leaving the dialyzer was higher than that entering, *Salvadeo* et al. [24] were unable to detect a change. However, *Salvadeo* and coworkers were able to detect a decrease in the aluminum concentration in the dialysate leaving the dialyzers when compared with that entering. *Salvadeo* et al. [24] did not mention the studies of either *Kaehny* et al. [14] or *Kovalchik* et al. [18] and failed to offer some explanation for the contrasting findings.

Allain et al. [3] obtained different results from both the work of *Kaehny* et al. [14] and ourselves [16]. These workers found that significant amounts of aluminum could be removed from plasma during dialysis against a dialysate containing only 10 μg/l of aluminum. However, *Allain* et al. [3] did observe plasma loading with aluminum in patients dialyzed against a high aluminum containing dialysate.

Gorsky and Dietz [9] obtained similar inconsistent results in a study of 21 patients where blood was analyzed both before and after dialysis. 10 of the patients had increased serum aluminum concentrations after dialysis, and 11 patients showed decreased concentrations. The observation of an increase or decrease was not apparently related to the serum aluminum concentrations which ranged from 27 to 254 μg/l. Isolated ultrafiltration removed part of the serum aluminum, but most remained bound to a nonfiltrable component.

Graf et al. [10, 11] studied aluminum kinetics in 24 patients on chronic hemodialysis. All patients had elevated predialysis serum aluminum concentrations (mean ~ 93 μg/l). When dialysis solutions with very low aluminum concentrations were used (2.7−8.1 μg/l), there were significant decreases of plasma aluminum during dialyzer passage. The mean aluminum concentration at the dialyzer blood inflow was 86 ± 36 μg/l which decreased to 72 ± 34 μg/l at the blood outflow site 5 min after the start of hemodialysis. After 6 h of dialysis the plasma aluminum concentrations were significantly lower ($p > 0.001$) than the predialysis values as demonstrated by a mean concentration of 57 ± 34 μg/l. These workers also measured an in vivo ultrafiltrable aluminum concentration by disconnecting the dialysate supply from the dialyzer and applying a reduced pressure of 200 mm/Hg using a suction pump to obtain 16 ml of ultrafiltrate. They obtained ultrafiltrate values of 18 ± 7 μg/l (20% of total aluminum) which were well in excess of the dialysate aluminum concentration. These workers concluded that the driving force for aluminum transfer was the effective concentration gradient between dialysate aluminum and the free diffusible plasma aluminum concentration. Moreover, they attributed any hyperaluminemia in their patients to factors other than aluminum loading during dialysis, with enhanced gastrointestinal absorption being the obvious major source.

One other factor to consider is that the removal of plasma aluminum during hemodialysis with a dialysate of low aluminum content may be associated with dialysate pH. *Gacek* et al. [8] have shown that due to the amphoteric nature of aluminum a highly water-insoluble aluminum hydroxide is formed near neutral pH. A small change in pH, either to a more acid or alkaline value, can make a large difference in the amount of aluminum in the dialyzable form. The final pH value of the dialysate can be affected by the pH of the water used to reconstitute the dialysate. Therefore, the pH of the dialysate can vary among dialysis centers due to the large variation in tap water pH in the USA, and this variation may have played some role in producing the conflicting reports concerning aluminum transfer across the membrane during hemodialysis.

The chemical properties of Al (III) have been studied; however, the complexation behavior of Al (III) with chelating or complexing agents has been ambiguous because a polymerization characteristic to Al (III) has restricted a detailed investigation. Some detailed information on the physicochemical stability of Al (III) in pharmaceutical phosphate buffer solutions has been reported by *Hasegawa* et al. [12, 13]. In general, carboxylic acids such as citric, glycolic, lactic, malic, malonic, oxalic, and amino acids, etc. complexed Al (III) more strongly at pH values close to their pKa values. It was concluded the pH of the solutions should be selected carefully for physicochemically stable parenteral foundations. The complexes of Al (III) with citric acid in phosphate buffer solutions were studied by gel filtration [13] and emphasized the marked effect of changes in pH values on the nature of any Al (III) complex with phosphate, carboxylic acid, and chelating agents.

Parkinson et al. [22] recognized the effect of controlling the dialysate pH to close to 7.0 to keep the aluminum in a colloidal form. The importance of dialysis fluid pH is emphasized in a report by *Branger* et al. [4] using the Redy system of dialysate regeneration which releases more aluminum from the cartridge when used with bicarbonate-containing dialysis fluid than with the usual acetate solution. *Parkinson* et al. [22] pointed out that most studies of aluminum transfer during dialysis show a rapid uptake by the blood, unless the dialysate aluminum concentration is kept down to about 10 μg/l [14, 18, 26]. At this concentration which uses water purified by reverse osmosis, a zero aluminum balance across the dialyzer can be achieved. The results of *Graf* et al. [10, 11], where aluminum removal was observed, possibly were due to the use of very pure water and also in part to the fact that the patients undergoing treatment had higher initial serum aluminum concentrations. Similarly *O'Hare and Murnaghan* [20] demonstrated a reduction in serum aluminum concentrations in 15 patients on chronic hemodialysis from 454 ± 191 to 273 ± 117 μ/l over a 9-month period. The water used to prepare the dialysate had an aluminum concentration consistently less than 10 μg/l. The major emphasis of this study was on the reversal of aluminum-induced hemodialysis anemia which is a microcytic anemia not due to iron deficiency. *Elliott and MacDougall* [5] were the first to observe a severe anemia preceding dialysis encephalopathy and vitamin D resistant dialysis osteomalacia. In the study of *O'Hare and Murnaghan* [20] there was an improvement in the anemia in the patients studied which coincided with a slow but substantial fall in serum aluminum concentration.

It does appear from the varying reports that the transfer of aluminum during dialysis is dependent to some extent on pH value and aluminum concentration of the dialysis solution and on the aluminum concentration of the serum, especially the ultrafiltrable fraction.

Concluding Remarks

It is now recognized, for patients maintained on intermittent hemodialysis, that the water used to prepare the dialysate fluid is potentially the most important source of aluminum.

Transfer of aluminum from the dialysate across the dialysis membrane into the patient's bloodstream during hemodialysis appears to occur unless the aluminum content of the dialysate is extremely low; there are reports of aluminum transfer at concentrations below 10 µg/l. At this latter level, however, there are conflicting reports regarding aluminum transfer across the dialysis membrane from the dialysate to the patient. Some laboratories have reported consistent loading, even at serum aluminum concentrations below 10 µg/l. Others have reported removal of aluminum from blood at these low concentrations, especially when dealing with patients with high total serum aluminum and high diffusible (or ultrafiltrable) aluminum concentrations. Some workers have reported both losses and uptake of aluminum in their patients. Overall, however, most of the information available indicates that zero aluminum balance across the dialyzer can be achieved at a dialysate aluminum concentration close to 10 µg/l. Some of the conflicting data in the literature might be due to the complex nature of aluminum species in water. Small changes in the dialysate pH can change the aluminum from a highly insoluble colloidal form to much more water-soluble species. Aluminum is amphoteric, and the insoluble form predominates at neutral pH, whereas a small change in pH to either a more acid or alkali value can make a large difference in the amount of aluminum in the dialyzable form. It appears that a dialysate pH of 7.4 is desirable in order to minimize transfer of aluminum across the membrane.

One area of considerable importance in obtaining a better understanding of such aluminum transfer involves the distribution of aluminum in plasma. Most reports consistently find that aluminum is partly protein bound and partly bound to lower molecular weight compounds (ultrafiltrable). Resolution of such binding species has been accomplished by gel filtration chromatography. However, identification of such species has not been made and is the next obvious area of investigation. Also distribution patterns in a wide variety of samples from normals and patients on intermittent hemodialysis with varying degrees of hyperaluminumia are needed. In addition, distribution patterns during treatment with chelating agents would provide interesting results. Gel filtration is a tedious procedure, and the next refinement of the separation technique almost certainly will involve high-performance liquid chromatography with the molecular exclusion columns. These techniques provide rapid separations on small quantities of sample and are ideally suited to studies on the distribution of aluminum in blood and tissues.

Information obtained using these techniques will help to elucidate the mechanism(s) by which aluminum manifests its toxic effects.

References

1   Alfrey, A.C.: Dialysis encephalopathy syndrome. A. Rev. Med. *29*: 93−98 (1978).
2   Alfrey, A.C.; LeGendre, G.R.; Kaehny, W.D.: The dialysis encephalopathy syndrome. Possible aluminum intoxication. New Engl. J. Med. *294*: 184−188 (1976).
3   Allain, P.; Thebaud, H.W.; Dupouet, L., et al.: Study of blood levels of a number of metals (Al, Mn, Cd, Pb, Cu, Zn) in chronic hemodialysis patients before and after dialysis. Nouv. Presse méd. *7*: 92 (1978).
4   Branger, B.; Ramperez, P.; Marigliano, N., et al.: Aluminium transfer in bicarbonate dialysis using a sorbent regeneration system: an in vitro study. Proc. Eur. Dial. Transplant Ass. *17*: 213−218 (1980).
5   Elliott, H.L.; MacDougall, A.L.: Aluminium studies in dialysis encephalopathy. Proc. Eur. Dial. Transplant Ass. *15*: 157−163 (1978).
6   Elliott, H.L.; MacDougall, A.I.; Fell, G.S.: Aluminum toxicity syndrome. Lancet *ii*: 1203 (1978).
7   Elliott, H.L.; MacDougall, A.I.; Fell, G.S., et al.: Plasmaphereses, aluminum and dialysis dementia. Lancet *ii*: 1255 (1978).
8   Gacek, E.M.; Babb, A.L.; Urelli, D.A., et al.: Dialysis dementia: the role of dialysate pH in altering the dializability of aluminum. Trans. Am. Soc. artif. internal Organs *25*: 409 (1979).
9   Gorsky, J.E.; Dietz, A.A.: Aluminium concentrations in serum of hemodialysis patients. Clin. Chem. *27*: 932−935 (1981).
10 Graf, H.; Stummvoll, H.K.; Meisinger, V.: Dialysate aluminum concentration and aluminum transfer during haemodialysis. Lancet *ii*: 46−47 (1982).
11 Graf, H.; Stummvoll, H.K.; Meisinger, V., et al.: Aluminum removal by hemodialysis. Kidney int. *19*: 587−592 (1981).
12 Hasegawa, K.; Hashi, K.; Okada, R.: Physicochemical stability of pharmaceutical phosphate buffer solutions. II. Complexation behavior of Al(III) with additives in phosphate buffer solutions. J. parenteral Sci. Tech. *36*: 168−173 (1982).
13 Hasegawa, K.; Hashi, K.; Okada, R.: III. Gel filtration chromatography of Al(III) complex formed in phosphate buffer. J. parenteral Sci. Tech. *36*: 174−178 (1982).
14 Kaehny, W.D.; Alfrey, A.C.; Holman, R.E., et al.: Aluminium transfer during hemodialysis. Kidney int. *12*: 361 (1977).
15 Kaehny, W.D.; Hegg, A.P.; Alfrey, A.C.: Gastrointestinal absorption of aluminum from aluminum-containing antacids. New Engl. J. Med. *296*: 1389−1390 (1977).
16 King, S.W.; Savory, J.; Wills, M.R.: Aluminium distribution in serum following hemodialysis. Ann. clin. Lab. Sci. *12*: 143−149 (1982).

17 King, S.W.; Wills, M.R.; Savory, J.: Serum binding of aluminium. Res. Commun. chem. Pathol. Pharmacol. *26*: 161–169 (1979).
18 Kovalchik, M.T.; Kaehny, W.D.; Hegg, A.P., et al.: Aluminium kinetics during hemodialysis. J. Lab. clin. Med. *92*: 712–720 (1978).
19 Lundin, A.P.; Caruso, C.; Sass, M., et al.: Ultrafiltrable aluminum in serum of normal man (Abstract). Clin. Res. *26*: 636 (1978).
20 O'Hare, J.A.; Murnaghan, D.J.: Reversal of aluminum-induced hemodialysis anemia by a low-aluminum dialysate. New Engl. J. Med. *306*: 654–656 (1982).
21 Parkinson, I.S.; Ward, M.K.; Feest, T.G., et al.: Fracturing dialysis osteodystrophy and dialysis encephalopathy. An epidemiological survey. Lancet *i*: 406–409 (1979).
22 Parkinson, I.S.; Ward, M.K.; Kerr, D.N.S.: Dialysis encephalopathy, bone disease and anaemia· the aluminum intoxication syndrome during regular haemodialysis. J. clin. Path. *34*: 1284–1285 (1981).
23 Recker, R.R.; Blotcky, A.J.; Leffler, J.A., et al.: Evidence for aluminum absorption from the gastrointestinal tract and bone deposition by aluminum carbonate ingestion with normal renal function. J. Lab. clin. Med. *90*: 810–815 (1977).
24 Salvadeo, A.; Minoia, C.; Segagni, S., et al.: Trace metal changes in dialysis fluid and blood of patients on hemodialysis. Int. J. artif. Organs *2*: 17 (1979).
25 Toffaletti, J.; Savory, J.; Gitelman, H.J.: Use of gel filtration to examine the distribution of calcium among serum proteins. Clin. Chem. *23*: 2306–2310 (1977).
26 Tsukamoto, Y.; Iwanami, S.; Marumo, F.: Disturbances of trace element concentrations in plasma of patients with chronic renal failure. Nephron *26*: 174–179 (1980).

J. Savory, PhD, Departments of Pathology, Biochemistry, University of
Virginia Medical Center, Charlottesville, VA 22908 (USA)

Contr. Nephrol., vol. 38, pp. 24–31 (Karger, Basel 1984)

Gastrointestinal Absorption of Aluminium in Chronic Renal Insufficiency

O. Knoll, H. Kellinghaus, H.P. Bertram, H. Zumkley, U. Graefe

Medizinische Poliklinik, Münster, FRG

Introduction

In 1976 when aluminium (Al) was identified as the aetiological factor of progressive dialysis encephalopathy (DE), two possible routes of intoxication were discussed. Intoxication of the *dialysis water* could explain the high incidence of DE in areas with a high Al concentration in the tap water, in countries using untreated water for the preparation of the bath and in hospitals with water supplies releasing Al [8, 9, 15, 16]. The *oral route* became probable because of the following observations: (1) the first cases of DE were observed 2–3 years after the establishment of phosphate-binding therapy with Al hydroxide (Al [OH]$_3$) in clinical routine, haemodialysis had been performed about 10 years before without such complications [1]; (2) typical courses of DE were seen in patients dialysed with Al-free water [1, 6, 12–14], and (3) a few cases of DE were seen in patients with chronic renal failure (CRF) in the predialytic state and therefore not yet in contact with Al-contaminated baths [12, 15].

This article reports our own data obtained from healthy volunteers and renal patients and reviews published investigations on the gastrointestinal absorption of Al compounds.

Clinical investigations were hindered by several factors. So in most patients on regular dialysis treatment (RDT) both routes of Al intoxication had to be considered, since the water used for the bath preparation was Al-contaminated and patients were treated additionally with Al (OH)$_3$. Therefore only patients in the predialytic state and patients using reverse osmosis for water preparation will be included in the following.

Another factor impeding clinical investigations is the lack of a sensitive and valid indicator of Al body burden. The syndrome DE is a rare disease, therefore in most studies only a few patients could be analysed. The Al serum level, however, is not well correlated with tissue concentrations. Al shifts from tissue to serum compartments and vice versa have been observed under several clinical conditions [1, 4, 5, 15, 16]. Analysis of tissue concentrations cannot be done repeatedly in renal patients for ethical reasons, however.

Al Sources for Oral Ingestion

Al $(OH)_3$ and several other Al-containing phosphate-binding agents and antacids are the most important sources of Al for renal patients. Al-containing resins are less important. Most patients suffering from CRF in the predialytic or even dialytic state need Al $(OH)_3$ or other Al compounds for withdrawal of alimentary phosphate and therewith for prophylaxis of secondary hyperparathyroidism. Dietary restrictions and phosphate elimination by dialysis are insufficient for controlling phosphate balance in most cases. In most patients on RDT the daily intake is within the range of 2.5–10.0 g Al $(OH)_3$ days i.e. 0.8–3.5 g Al/day. The Al content of food and drinking water may be neglected, since even in the case of extreme Al contamination (cooking in Al pots, many wines, etc.) oral ingestion will not exceed a few milligrams daily.

Principles of Al Absorption

In former years Al compounds used as antacids or as phosphate-binding agents were thought not to be absorbed but excreted completely with the faeces. In 1970, *Berlyne* et al. [2] were the first to make Al absorption and accumulation in renal patients probable. The development of highly sensitive analytic techniques, especially flameless atomic absorption spectrophotometry, made the examination of Al absorption possible in the last decade. It is supposed that only Al ions are able to cross the mucosa barrier in the gastrointestinal tract. Therefore the absorption rate depends essentially on the ionised Al fraction [4, 8, 10, 13, 14]. Al-containing phosphate binders and antacids react as amphoterics: solubility increases with low pH as with high pH, whereas these compounds are not ionised as colloids in a neutral pH range. *Gacek* et al. [8] demonstrated in an in vitro study that ionisation and solubility of Al $(OH)_3$ increase with a pH shift of one unit below pH 6.5 by the factor 100,000. This means that the solubility and absorption rate depend much more on the pH of the gastrointestinal tract than on the Al $(OH)_3$ intake. Great variability of gastrointestinal pH must cause great individual variability of Al absorption. The intake of phosphate-binding agents with the food as recommended improves not only phosphate withdrawal but diminishes the possibly ionised Al fraction by buffering the acidic stomach pH with the food. The intake of Al $(OH)_3$ without food is not useful for phosphate binding but also increases the ionised Al fraction and possibly the absorption rate, since stomach pH is extremely low. On the other hand, *Clarkson* et al. [4] found no relation between Al balance and pentagastrin-stimulated secretion.

Several clinical studies revealed different Al absorption from different Al compounds [3, 10, 13]. Possibly due to individual variability and to the low number of cases, the reproducibility of the findings was not sufficient and the results are controversial. Concentrations of other ions influence solubility and absorption of Al compounds, too. So Al phosphate was found insoluble, whereas Al fluoride was absorbed to an high extent [10]. By this way, the absorption rate of Al-containing drugs depends not only on the gastrointestinal pH, but also on the contents of food and other drugs ingested simultaneously. Moreover, influences of parathyroid hormone on Al absorption were supposed. Increased Al toxicity in hyperparathyroidism might also be due to Al mobilisation from bone depots. Other clinical studies revealed suppressed activity of parathyroid hormone in hyperaluminaemia. In summary interactions between parathyroid hormone and Al distribution and absorption must be assumed, but are not sufficiently analysed [4, 5, 15, 16]. Uremic lesions of gastrointestinal mucosa cells might influence trace metal absorption too, as is known from food contents.

Al Absorption in Subjects with Normal Renal Function

Systemic Al intoxications have been seen in patients with impaired renal function, in most cases in patients on RDT. So normal excretory renal function was supposed to be sufficient for avoiding critical Al overload. Though many patients suffering from gastric or duodenal ulcers are treated with high doses of Al-containing antacids over many months or even years, no case of DE was described in those patients. It was assumed that in healthy subjects Al is not absorbed from the gastrointestinal tract. *Zumkley* et al. [17] found increasing Al plasma levels under treatment with magnesium

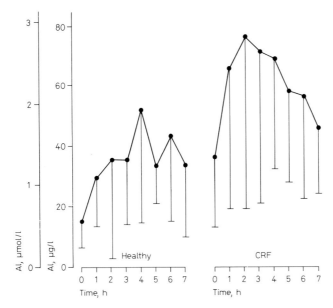

Fig. 1. Serum aluminium (Al) levels after ingestion of 2,400 mg Al (OH)$_3$ (time 0) in 13 healthy volunteers and in 19 patients with predialytic chronic renal failure (CRF), admitted for fistula surgery (mean − 1 SD).

and Al-containing antacids only in patients with CRF. On the other hand *Kaehny* et al. [10] and *Bertram und Zumkley* [3] observed a marked increase of Al serum concentration after a single dose of Al (OH)$_3$ and other compounds in healthy volunteers.

In our own study, Al serum levels and urinary excretion were measured in 13 healthy volunteers. A marked increase of serum levels occurred 1−6 h after ingestion of a single dose of 2.4 g Al (OH)$_3$ (fig. 1). Differences in the peak amplitude and the peak latency were not significant after ingestion of different phosphate-binding agents. Urinary excretion of Al was raised even on the 4th day after ingestion of the antacid (fig. 2). There is no doubt that Al is absorbed from antacids in healthy subjects, too. Prolonged renal excretion makes accumulation of the trace metal probable.

Al Absorption in Predialytic State of CRF

In patients suffering from CRF not yet requiring RDT, Al accumulation is facilitated by the oral intake of phosphate-binding agents and by im-

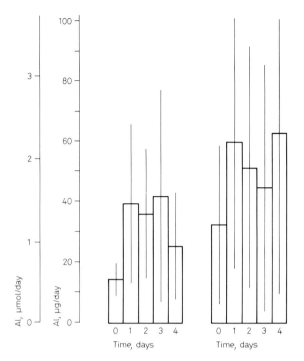

Fig. 2. Urinary aluminium (Al) excretion before (0) and on days 1, 2, 3 and 4 after ingestion of 2,400 mg Al (OH)$_3$ in 13 healthy volunteers and in 19 patients with predialytic chronic renal failure (CRF), admitted for fistula surgery (mean ± 1 SD).

paired renal Al excretion. Al clearances were found less than creatinine clearance [2, 10]. Several cases of typical DE due to Al accumulation have been published [15]. Essentially raised Al serum levels were found in patients with CRF treated with Al-containing compounds [1, 2, 4, 7, 11, 12, 18]. Serum levels were significantly higher in CRF patients on Al (OH)$_3$ than in patients not on treatment with phosphate-binding agents [11, 18]. In our own study, Al absorption was examined in patients admitted for shunt surgery. Pre-treatment Al serum levels were higher than in healthy volunteers, although patients were not on treatment with Al-containing drugs before (fig. 1). This difference must be due to reduced renal excretion of Al ingested with food and drinking water. Peak levels of Al serum concentration were obtained 1–5 h after ingestion of a single dose of 2.4 g Al (OH)$_3$. Ingestion of different phosphate-binding agents induced similar changes of serum level. Urinary excretion was high even on the 4th day

Table I. Incidence of progressive dialysis encephalopathy (DE), deterioration of renal anaemia (An) and symptomatic bone disease (BD) in patients on regular haemodialysis treatment

Aluminium		n	DE		An		BD	
µg/l	µmol/l		n	%	n	%	n	%
Softener								
<100	< 3.7	25	–	–	–	–	2	8
100–200	3.7– 7.4	42	–	–	2	4.8	5	11.9
200–300	7.4–11.1	12	–	–	1	8.3	5	41.7
>300	>11.1	4	3	75	4	100	4	100
Reverse osmosis								
<100	< 3.7	23	–	–	–	–	2	8.7
100–200	3.7– 7.4	4	–	–	–	–	1	25
200–300	7.4–11.1	2	2	100	2	100	2	100
>300	>11.1	2	–	–	2	100	2	100

Deterioration of anaemia was valued, if a haematocrit fall of more than 5 percent was not explained by blood loss, iron deficiency or inadequate dialysis. Symptomatic bone disease was valued in any case suffering from pain or fractures regardless of chemical, radiological and histological findings. Incidence of clinical symptoms was related to the mode of water preparation (softener or reverse osmosis) and to aluminium plasma levels.

after intake of the drug (fig. 2). Al accumulation is facilitated in these patients by decreasing Al clearance.

Al Absorption in Patients on RDT

In the publication by *Alfrey* et al. [1] in 1976, in which Al was identified as aetiological factor of DE, a significant dependence of the Al tissue concentration on the time on RDT, in this case identical with the time on Al $(OH)_3$, was described. If dialysis water was in fact nearly free of Al, this finding confirms the role of oral Al for intoxication. Generally Al serum levels were higher in dialysis patients on Al $(OH)_3$ than in patients without phosphate-binding therapy [6, 9, 12–16, 18]. In patients using reverse osmosis water for preparation of the bath, a correlation between the daily intake of Al $(OH)_3$ and Al serum levels was found significant by several investigators, but not by others [9, 13]. Different results may be due partly to the different Al absorption of patients, to the different time on RDT or phosphate-binding therapy, or to the differences of trace metal distribution in body compartments. But undoubtedly reduction of the daily intake of Al-containing phosphate-binding agents is able to lower Al serum levels [6, 13–15].

In our own evaluation of patients on home haemodialysis or on limited care haemodialysis, high Al serum levels were less frequent in the group using reverse osmosis for water preparation than in those patients using softeners (table I). But in patients using Al-free reverse osmosis water, extreme Al levels were also found. The clinical consequences of Al intoxication (DE, deterioration of renal anaemia, osteomalacic bone disease) were seen in both groups of patients.

In conclusion there are enough clinical data obtained from patients dialysed with Al-free water to confirm the essential role of oral Al intake for the critical accumulation of the trace metal. Al absorption was investigated preferentially in patients with CRF in the predialytic state because, in these patients, the influences of dialysis on Al balance can be excluded. Al-containing phosphate-binding agents are furthermore necessary for the prophylaxis of secondary hyperparathyroidism and extraosseous calcifications, but strict dietary restrictions, the use of dialysers providing high phosphate clearance and, in some cases, higher dialysis frequency are able to lower the risk of Al intoxication essentially, if the dialysis water is not Al-contaminated.

References

1   Alfrey, A.C.; LeGendre, G.R.; Kaehny, W.D.: The dialysis encephalopathy syndrome. Possible aluminium intoxication. New Engl. J. Med. *294*: 184–188 (1976).

2   Berlyne, G.M.; Pest, D.; Ben Ari, J.; Weinberger, J.; Stern, M.; Gilmore, G.R.; Levine, R.: Hyperaluminaemia from aluminium resins in renal failure. Lancet *ii*: 494–496 (1970).

3   Bertram, H.P.; Zumkley, H.: Magnesium- und Aluminiumresorption bei Behandlung mit Antazida. Krankenhausarzt *52*: 416–424 (1979).

4   Clarkson, E.M.; Luck, V.A.; Hynson, W.V.; Bailey, R.R.; Eastwood, J.B.; Woodhead, J.S.; Clements, V.R.; O'Riordan, J.L.H.; De Wardener, H.E.: The effect of aluminium hydroxide on calcium, phosphorus and aluminium balances, the serum parathyroid hormone concentration and the aluminium content of bone in patients with chronic renal failure. Clin. Sci. *43*: 519–531 (1972).

5   Drüeke, T.: Dialysis osteomalacia and aluminium intoxication. Nephron *26*: 207–210 (1980).

6   Fleming, L.W.; Stewart, W.K.; Fell, G.S.; Halls, D.J.: The effect of oral aluminium therapy on plasma aluminium levels in patients with chronic renal failure in an area with low water aluminium. Clin. Nephrol. *17*: 222–227 (1982).

7   Fuchs, C.; Brasche, M.; Donath, U.; Henning, H.V.; Knoll, D.; Nordbeck, H.; Paschen, K.; Quellhorst, E.; Scheler, F: Flammenlose Atomabsorption zur Spurenelementanalyse in biologischen Materialien – Aluminiumbestimmungen nach Aludroxgabe bei Niereninsuffizienz. Verh. dt. Ges. inn. Med. *79*: 683–685 (1973).

8   Gacek, E.M.; Babb, A.L.; Uvelli, D.A.; Fry, D.L.; Scribner, B.H.: Dialysis dementia: the role of dialysate pH in altering the dialyzability of aluminum. Trans. Am. Soc. artif. internal Organs *25*: 409–415 (1979).

9   Graefe, U.: Wasseraufbereitung und Aluminiumhaushalt. Nieren-Hochdruckkrankh. *10*: 217–220 (1981).

10   Kaehny, W.D.; Hegg, A.P.; Alfrey, A.C.: Gastrointestinal absorption of aluminum from aluminum-containing antacids. New Engl. J. Med. *296*: 1389–1391 (1977).

11   Marsden, S.N.E.; Parkinson, I.S.; Ward, M.K.; Ellis, H.A.; Kerr, D.N.S.: Evidence for aluminium accumulation in renal failure. Proc. Eur. Dial. Transplant Ass. *16*: 588–595 (1979).

12   McKinney, T.D.; Basinger, M.; Dawson, E.; Jones, M.M.: Serum aluminum levels in dialysis dementia. Nephron *32*: 53–56 (1982).

13   Pogglitsch, H.: Therapie mit aluminiumhaltigen Substanzen in der Nephrologie. Nieren-Hochdruckkrankh. *10*: 210–216 (1981).

14   Pogglitsch, H.; Wawschinek, O.; Holzer, H.; Petek, W.; Katschnig, H.; Ladurner, G.: Beziehungen zwischen Plasmaaluminium, peroraler Aluminiumhydroxydaufnahme und Enzephalopathiesymptomen bei Dauerdialysepatienten. Nieren-Hochdruckkrankh. *9*: 284–289 (1980).

15   Sideman, S.; Manor, D.: The dialysis dementia syndrome and aluminum intoxication. Nephron. *31*: 1–10 (1982).

16   Ward, M.K.; Pierides, A.M.; Fawcett, P.; Shaw, D.A.; Perry, R.H.; Tomlinson, B.E.; Kerr, D.N.S.: Dialysis encephalopathy syndrome. Proc. Eur. Dial. Transplant Ass. *13*: 348–354 (1976).

17   Zumkley, H.; Bertram, H.P.; Lison, A.; Ernst, M.: Oral administration of magnesium and aluminium during renal insufficiency; in Hemphill, Trace substances in environmental health (Columbia University Press, New York 1978).

18   Zumkley, H.; Bertram, H.P.; Lison, A.; Knoll, O.; Losse, H.: Aluminium, zinc and copper concentrations in plasma in chronic renal insufficiency. Clin. Nephrol. *12*: 18–21 (1979).

Priv.-Doz. Dr. O. Knoll, Medizinische Poliklinik, Domagkstrasse 3,
D-4400 Münster (FRG)

Contr. Nephrol., vol. 38, pp. 32−36 (Karger, Basel 1984)

Aluminum-Free Intestinal Phosphate Binding

H. Schneider, K.D. Kulbe, H. Weber, E. Streicher

Katharinenhospital and Fraunhofer Institute for Interfacial and Bioengineering Sciences, Stuttgart, FRG

Aluminum accumulation and its sequelae in chronic renal failure patients [1−3] are possibly a consequence of aluminum hydroxide medication, as far as correct water preparation for dialysis is guaranteed. For the purpose of intestinal phosphate binding we developed aluminum-free substances which were tested in vitro and in vivo.

Methods

The substances tested consisted of 1- to 2-mm particles of natural polymers charged with calcium or a combination of calcium and iron (Fe^{++} and Fe^{+++}). This group of substances is nontoxic and does not cause constipation. We studied the in vitro capacity of phosphate removal in Tris buffer solution under different pH conditions. Furthermore the substance was incubated with human duodenal juice, which was enriched with 2g sodium phosphate imitating the phosphate load of an average meal. During the 2−hour incubation period the phosphate binding capacity was determined.

10 chronic renal failure patients with recurrent problems controlling their serum phosphate levels by conventional aluminum hydroxide therapy were treated with the calcium-charged substance for 4 weeks to 3 months.

Results

The polymer charged with calcium or a combination of calcium and iron contained small amounts of sodium (20 mg/g) and potassium (7.8 mg/g). The calcium content was found to be 140−160 mg/g, the iron content of the calcium-iron-charged product was 40 mg/g (fig. 1).

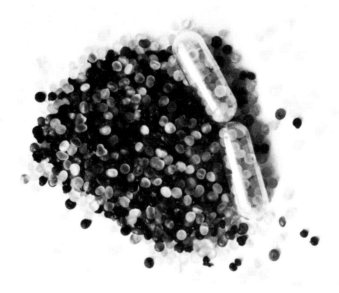

Fig. 1. Mixture of the polymeric substance. Light particles are calcium-charged, dark particles are charged with a combination of calcium and iron.

1 g substance was incubated in 200 ml Tris-bufferred solution which contained 0.4 g phosphate (fig. 2). The calcium-charged substance failed to work under acidotic pH conditions (pH 2), whereas the calcium-iron-charged product was capable of binding 0.05 g phosphate (16% of total binding capacity) under acidotic conditions. Coming to neutral and alkalotic pH values, the particles swelled allowing phosphate to be entrapped. The calcium-charged substance was capable of binding 0.2 g phosphate (50%), whereas the calcium-iron-charged product neutralized 0.29 g phosphate (72.5%) in comparison to Aludrox®, which just bound 0.095 g phosphate (23.75%) under these conditions.

To obtain a test procedure a little closer to the physiologic conditions we chose human duodenal juice enriched with 2 g sodium phosphate (fig. 3). This solution was incubated with 2.4 g calcium-charged phosphate binder and stirred at 37°C. During the first 45 min a sharp decline of the phosphate concentration was noted followed by only minor changes for the rest of the incubation time. After 120 min phosphate concentrations close to those found prior to the phosphate load were reached.

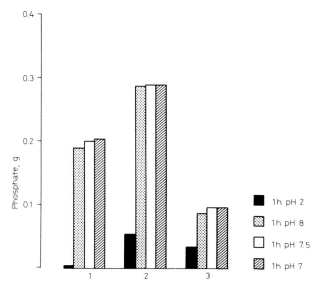

Fig. 2. Phosphate binding capacity (per gram substance) of the calcium-charged product (1) and the calcium-iron-charged polymer (2) in comparison with Aludrox® (3) under different pH conditions.

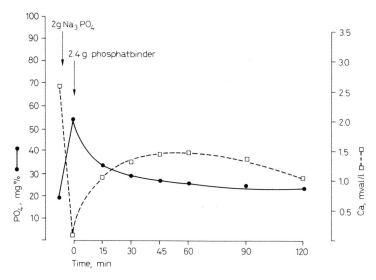

Fig. 3. Phosphate binding effect of 2.4 g calcium-charged polymer in 500 ml human duodenal juice at 37°C (pH 7−8) enriched with 2 g sodium phosphate over a 120-min incubation period.

Table I. Mean serum phosphate, serum calcium and serum potassium levels of 10 chronic renal failure patients on hemodialysis treated with the calcium-charged polymer at a dosage of 4−7 g/day

	Before treatment	After 4 weeks of treatment	After 8 weeks of treatment
Serum phosphate mg%	8.5 ± 1.7	6.0 ± 2.0	5.5 ± 1.1
Serum calcium mmol/l	2.35 ± 0.23	2.44 ± 0.21	2.41 ± 0.16
Serum potassium mmol/l	5.7 ± 0.6	5.4 ± 0.7	5.1 ± 0.4

10 patients suffering from end-stage renal failure on hemodialysis with permanently elevated serum phosphate levels despite conventional aluminum hydroxide therapy were treated with the calcium-charged product for 4 weeks to 3 months (table I). We did not detect undesirable side effects, and constipation, a frequent problem under aluminum hydroxide therapy, was minimized. With a dose of 4−7 g/day serum phosphate levels dropped from 8.5 ± 1.7 to 5.5 ± 1.1 mg%, whereas serum calcium levels increased slightly from 2.35 ± 0.23 to 2.41 ± 0.16 mmol/l. Serum potassium values decreased from 5.7 ± 0.6 to 5.1 ± 0.4 mmol/l.

Discussion

According to the EDTA Registry [4] over 90% of dialysis centers regularly give aluminum-containing phosphate binders to some or all of their patients. Only a minority of centers (16%) regularly monitor aluminum levels in water and dialysis fluid and in patients' serum [4], so that the question as to the cause of aluminum accumulation cannot be answered reliably at the moment. There is evidence to suggest [3] that aluminum is resorbed enterally; it should therefore be abandoned if possible.

The new substances tested for their phosphate binding capacity are made of natural polymers and charged with calcium and iron cations. Whereas the iron-containing preparation already trapped phosphate under acidotic pH conditions, neutral alkalotic pH values caused the particles to swell and dissolve in the presence of phosphate. Calcium was released gradually and calcium phosphate was formed. The calcium phosphate thus formed partially adhered to the polymeric matrix. Depending on the polymer's calcium load and the phosphate ingestion there might be a reasonable amount of calcium available for resorption, as serum calcium values rose in some patients. Possibly a cation exchange between calcium or sodium and potassium also took place, as we noticed decreasing serum potassium levels. As far as the in vitro experiments are concerned, the phosphate binding efficacy per gram substance was 2–3 times higher than it was for Aludrox®. This polymer system can also be used for controlled release of other ions (e.g. zinc, magnesium) and of water-soluble drugs avoiding undesirably high substance concentrations.

References

1   Alfrey, A.C.; Mishell, J.M.; Burks, J.; Contiguglia, S.R.; Rudolph, H.; Lewin, E.; Holmes, J.H.: Syndrome of dyspraxia and multifocal seizures associated with chronic hemodialysis. Trans. Am. Soc. artif. internal Organs *18*: 257–261 (1972).
2   Pierides, A.M.; Edwards, W.G.; Cullum, U.X.; McCall, J.T.; Ellis, H.A.: Hemodialysis encephalopathy with osteomalacic fractures and muscle weakness. Kidney int. *18*: 115–124 (1980).
3   Ulmer, D.D.: Toxicity from aluminium antacids. New Engl. J. Med. *294*: 218–219 (1976).
4   Wing, A.J.: Report of EDTA Registry on water preparation, dialysis practice and encephalopathy in dialysis patients in the European Community 1981. Int. Workshop on the Role of Biol. Monitoring in the Prevention of Aluminium Toxicity in Man, Luxembourg 1982.

Dr. H. Schneider, Department of Nephrology and Hypertension, Katharinenhospital, D-7000 Stuttgart (FRG)

Contr. Nephrol., vol. 38, pp. 37–46 (Karger, Basel 1984)

Correlation of Serum Aluminum Values with Tissue Aluminum Concentration

Marc E. De Broe[a], Frank L. Van de Vyver[a], Arline B. Bekaert[a], Patrick D'Haese[a], Guy J. Paulus[a], Walter J. Visser[b], René Van Grieken[a], Frederik A. de Wolff[c], Armand H. Verbueken[a]

[a]Department of Nephrology-Hypertension, Pathology and Chemistry, University of Antwerp, Belgium; [b]Department of Pathology, University of Utrecht, The Netherlands; [c]Laboratory of Toxicology, University of Leiden, The Netherlands

Introduction

Aluminum accumulates in the bodies of patients with severe renal failure [1], and patients being treated with chronic hemodialysis are more exposed to aluminum than any other patient group due to the aluminum in the dialysate and the orally administered aluminum in phosphate binders. This accumulation in the tissue sometimes results in bone disease such as osteomalacia [2] and damage to the brain leading to encephalopathy [3].

Although the exact toxicity mechanism in the bone remains to be determined, important information concerning the localization and concentration of aluminum in bone, and treatment of 'dialysis osteomalacia' [4] is available. Due to methodological problems, the information on 'aluminum brain damage' is scarce [5]. The nephrologist, aware of these two dramatic diseases, urgently needs simple reliable methods to enable him to make an early diagnosis of aluminum accumulation in his hemodialysis patients. Furthermore, if his patients have already been dialyzed for some years, he needs an appropriate treatment for those with an established heavy aluminum body burden.

In this contribution, we will discuss some information from the literature and some of our own results concerning the correlation of plasma aluminum values with tissue concentrations.

Materials and Methods

Serum and Tissue Samples

Plasma from 489 patients on chronic hemodialysis at ten hemodialysis centers in three countries was collected using appropriate materials. Plastic syringes (Sarstedt, Monovette) equipped with a Terumo needle No. 1938 (16G) were used, since it has been demonstrated that no aluminum was detected after a 5-day stagnation test. The samples were stored at 4 °C.

Transiliac bone biopsies were taken from dialyzed patients and patients with severe renal failure ± 2 cm beneath and dorsal to the anterior superior iliac spine with a trephine 7 mm in diameter (Bordier, Meunier). Histological investigation of the bone specimens was performed after 24 h fixation in *Burkhardt*'s [6] solution and transfer to absolute methanol. The specimens were embedded in methylmethacrylate and the undecalcified sections were cut from the biopsies with a Jung K sledge microtome. The serial sections (8 μm) were stained by means of Goldner's method for qualitative histology. An established histochemical method [7] using Aluminon (BDH Chemicals, UK) was used with slight modifications to detect aluminum in 8-μm undecalcified bone sections.

Liver biopsies were obtained with a Tru-cut® needle. The liver biopsies were treated with routine light and transmission electron microscopic procedures. The acid phosphatase reaction was performed according to *De Jong* et al. [8]. All biopsy material for aluminum assay was immediately weighed and aluminum was determined using atomic absorption spectrometry avoiding undesirable aluminum contamination. Some of the samples were assayed in two different laboratories (Leiden, Antwerp). For tissue preparation only plastic knives were used. The tissue was stored in polystyrene tubes with polyethylene caps (Biolab 898089).

For the destruction of tissue samples three methods were tested: Method 1, quartz Kjeldahl destruction with 5 ml HNO_3 (Merck suprapur); method 2, Uniseal decomposition vessel, destruction with 5 ml HNO_3 (Merck suprapur), 80 °C, 4h; method 3, quartz Kjeldahl destruction with a $HClO_4-H_2SO_4-HNO_3$ 1:1:3 mixture. Method 3 was rejected because the generated signal was unstable and the destruction was too aggressive for the apparatus. A recovery study carried out with methods 1 and 2 using aqueous standards yielded a recovery of 98–103%.

LAMMA is a recent mass spectrometric technique [9] consisting of a dual laser system and a time-of-flight mass spectrometer. Both lasers are focused together on a thin section of liver biopsy (0.2 μm) treated by the routine transmission electron microscopic procedure. The red low-energy He-Ne pilot laser selects the sites of analysis, while the high-power ultraviolet Nd-YAG Laser (266 nm) perforates the biological specimen. An area of a few square micrometers is evaporated and ionized and a complete mass spectrum is obtained for each laser shot. Transmission electron microscopy is used in combination with LAMMA to identify the type of analyzed material. For further description and application of this technique see *Schmidt* et al. [9] and *Van de Vyver* et al. [this vol.].

Results

The excellent correlation of plasma samples analyzed for aluminum in the two collaborating laboratories is shown in figure 1. The plasma

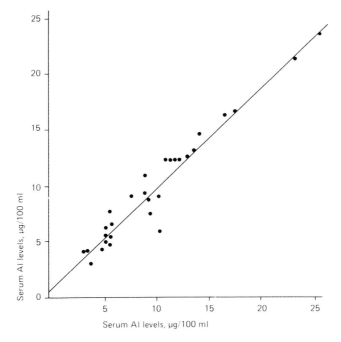

Fig. 1. Correlation between serum aluminum (μg/100 ml) measurements in laboratory 1 and laboratory 2.

aluminum levels of 489 patients with renal failure from ten hemodialysis centers are shown in figure 2. The plasma and bone tissue aluminum concentrations in patients with clinical, histological, and histochemical evidence of 'dialysis osteomalacia' compared to dialyzed patients without osteomalacia and normal controls are given in table I. In 2 out of 5 'dialyzed osteomalacia' patients, plasma aluminum levels below 70 μg/l were found. The bone tissue aluminum levels of the 'dialysis osteomalacia' patients, however, were found to be far in excess of those observed in dialysis patients without aluminum bone disease.

The tissue levels of aluminum in control patients and dialyzed patients are given in figure 3 and table II. The striking differences between the analyzed tissues, on the one hand, and the high aluminum concentration in the liver in the absence of clinical toxicity, on the other, led us to study the subcellular localization of aluminum in different tissues. LAMMA treatment of biopsy specimens of liver and bone of a patient with a large aluminum body burden demonstrated the presence of aluminum in elec-

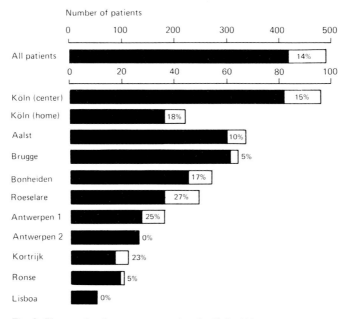

Fig. 2. Plasma aluminum concentration (µg/l) in 489 patients on hemodialysis. ■ = Below 100 µg/l; □ = in excess of 100 µg/l.

Table I. Patients with end-stage renal failure on chronic hemodialysis with aluminum osteomalacia

Patients	Age years	Sex	Months on dialysis	Aluminum levels		Osteomalacia in bone histology	Aluminum staining sections	Clinical toxicity
				plasma µg/l	bone µg/g = ppm			
D.S.G.	37	F	72	47	45	+	+	+
S.K.T.	52	M	43	1730	84	+	+	+
L.J.	40	F	96	62	25	+	+	+
C.A.	65	F	63	–	40	+	+	+
D.S.R.	44	M	54	378	100	+	+	+
Severe renal failure on dialysis				< 150	3	–	–	–
Controls				< 10	1			

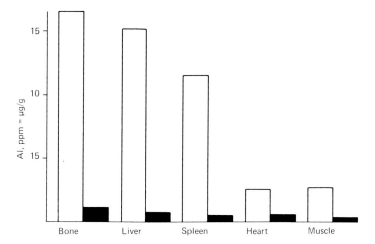

Fig. 3. Tissue aluminum levels. □ = Patients on chronic hemodialysis; ■ = control values.

Table II. Tissue aluminum levels in deceased chronic hemodialysis patients (ppm = μg/l)

	Mean ± SD	n
Bone	16.5 ± 11.9	9
Liver	15.2 ± 13.4	10
Spleen	11.5 ± 9.8	4
Heart	2.5 ± 1.8	6
Muscle	2.6 ± 1.4	9
Cerebellum		
White matter	6.4 ± 1.9	2
Gray matter	0.7 ± 0.4	4
Cerebrum		
White matter	0.6 ± 0.6	5
Gray matter	1.1 ± 0.9	6

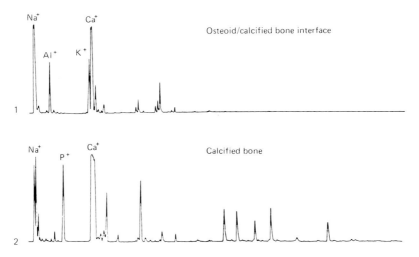

Fig. 4. LAMMA analysis of bone biopsies. An aluminum signal is observed at the osteoid/calcified-bone interface (1), but is absent at the level of calcified bone (2).

tron-dense bodies, which were identified as lysosomes upon histochemical reaction for acid phosphatase. The lysosomes of hepatocytes as well as Kupffer cells contained aluminum in the biopsy specimens studied. Using the LAMMA technique in bone, aluminum was demonstrated at the osteoid/calcified-bone interface. No aluminum signal was observed when calcified bone was studied (fig. 4).

Discussion

Contamination of samples with aluminum offers a major problem to the determination of aluminum levels in plasma or tissues. The nearly identical results obtained by two independent laboratories using slightly different atomic absorption spectrometric methods suggest the absence of contamination of our materials and the reliability of the results.

A multicenter study demonstrated that most chronic hemodialysis patients show plasma aluminum levels below 100 µg/l. However, a few exceptions were present in most centers. It should be noted that centers where dialysis therapy was started only recently and where reverse-osmosis water treatment is available show the lowest numbers of patients with plasma aluminum levels above 100 µg/l. This observation is consistent with the literature [10] and confirms that adequate dialysate water treatment is able to eliminate an important source of aluminum in hemodialysis patients.

Why does nearly every center have some patients with plasma aluminum levels above 100 µg/l despite adequate water purification? Probably other sources of aluminum, such as gastrointestinal aluminum absorption, play an important role in aluminum accumulation in end-stage renal failure patients whether or not they are treated with hemodialysis. Indeed, these patients receive significant amounts of aluminum, since most of them are treated orally with phosphate binders containing aluminum [11]. Individual factors increasing the ability to absorb aluminum from the gut are responsible for the observed differences in plasma concentration. Such factors may be of genetic origin and HLA-linked, as has been well documented for iron [12], or related to secondary hyperparathyroidism [13], which is frequently present in severe renal failure. The question of how far plasma aluminum is a reliable index for body burden of aluminum is still open. From our results, it is apparent that as far as patients with osteomalacia are concerned this certainly is not the case. In fact, 2 of 5 patients suffering from dialysis osteomalacia showed plasma aluminum levels below 100 µg/l. Other authors [14] have also reported similar plasma aluminum levels in some cases of proven dialysis osteomalacia. We may conclude that a plasma aluminum level below 100 µg/l does not exclude the presence of dialysis osteomalacia. The relative value of the aluminum concentration was again recently demonstrated by *Cannata* et al. [15]. These authors observed that increases in plasma aluminum returned to preload values 5–6 weeks after an acute exposure to an aluminum load in patients with continuous ambulatory peritoneal dialysis. This clearly shows that if determinations of plasma aluminum are performed at intervals of 4–6 months, acute loads with important tissue deposition will be missed.

The brain is another target of aluminum accumulation and this sometimes results in the dramatic clinical picture of encephalopathy. In 1976 *Alfrey* et al. [16] reported a substantial increase in the concentration of aluminum in several tissues of patients dying of encephalopathy. These results were confirmed by different groups [14, 17] (Eindhoven, Newcastle). In the United States, *Arieff* et al. [18] was reluctant to accept this evidence and claimed that he could not find a statistically significant difference in brain aluminum between patients in chronic renal failure without dialysis and patients with dialysis encephalopathy. The reason for this divergence could be that the brain aluminum concentration has traditionally been measured in the gray or white matter of the cerebrum. It could be that the aluminum level in other areas of the brain, such as the cerebellum, and even parts of it, is critical. In any way serum concentrations below 100 μg/l are observed in patients with dialysis encephalopathy [14].

We find that the subcellular localization of aluminum in bone and liver offers a considerable amount of information. In bone, aluminum was found at the osteoid/calcified-bone interface. Although the mechanisms by which aluminum interferes with normal bone mineralization are still unclear, its localization at this front forms an important indication that aluminum could interfere directly with the mineralization process. Further study is clearly needed to test this hypothesis.

Other theories such as interference with vitamin D metabolism [2] or an indirect effect of aluminum via a phosphate depletion syndrome [19] are less likely. The role of parathyroid hormone [20] in favoring abnormal aluminum accumulation in several tissues, including brain, bone, and parathyroid glands, has been demonstrated. In the liver, however, with equal or even higher concentrations of aluminum, no clinical evidence of toxicity has been observed. In the liver, the subcellular localization of aluminum in the lysosomes can be considered the most appropriate place to protect the cell from toxicity [21].

In conclusion, careful sampling avoiding contamination and accurate sensitive measurement are essential in the investigation of aluminum accumulation toxicity. Patients with proved aluminum osteomalacia may have a serum aluminum level below 100 μg/l. A single plasma aluminum determination cannot be used as a guide to previous exposure nor as a guide to the risk of clinical toxicity. The value of monitoring plasma aluminum levels in order to avoid aluminum accumulation toxicity remains to be determined. Bone tissue aluminum is elevated in patients with aluminum osteomalacia, and at present a bone biopsy specimen provides the best available information on the aluminum body burden, together with well-documented additional information on iron status and the presence of bone pathology. The subcellular localization of aluminum in different tissues contributes to the understanding of the described pathology in the bone and the absence of aluminum-related pathology in the liver.

Acknowledgement

We are most grateful to Dr. *J. Boelaert*, Dr. *V. Bosteels*, Dr. *M. Segaert*, Dr. *R. Lins*, Dr. *Lukowsky*, Dr. *Finke*, Dr. *G. Verpooten*, Dr. *D. Walb*, Dr. *J. Simoes* for referring their patients to us. We also thank the staffs and nursing teams of collaborating centers at Aalst

(Onze Lieve Vrouwziekenhuis), Antwerpen (Algemeen Ziekenhuis Stuivenberg, Kliniek Heilige Familie, Akademisch Ziekenhuis Antwerpen), Brugge (St. Janziekenhuis), Köln (Kuratorium für Heimdialyse und Transplantation, Merheim), Kortrijk (Kliniek Maria Voorzienigheid), Roeselare (Heilige Hartkliniek), Ronse (Zusters van Barmhartigheid), Brussel (UCL, St. Lucasziekenhuis), Lisboa (Santa Cruz). Last but not least our thanks are due to Mrs. *A. Grootveld* for secreterial help.

References

1   Alfrey, A.C.; Hegg, A.; Craswell, P.: Metabolism and toxicity of aluminium in renal failure. Am. J. clin. Nutr. *33*: 1509–1516 (1980).

2   Drueke, T.: Dialysis osteomalacia and aluminium intoxication. Nephron *26*: 207–210 (1980).

3   Dunea, G.; Mahurkar, S.D.; Mamdani, B.; Smith, E.C.: Role of aluminium in dialysis dementia. Ann. intern. Med. *88*: 502–504 (1978).

4   Hodsman, A.B.; Sherrard, D.J.; Wong, E.G.; Brickman, A.S.; Lee, D.B.N.; Alfrey, A.C.; Singer, F.R.; Norman, A.W.; Coburn, J.W.: Vitamin-D-resistant osteomalacia in hemodialysis patients lacking secondary hyperparathyroidism. Ann. intern. Med. *94*: 629–637 (1981).

5   Arieff, A.: Neurological complications of uremia; in Brenner, Rector, The kidney, pp. 2306–2343 (Saunders, Philadelphia 1981).

6   Burkhardt, R.: Präparative Voraussetzungen zur klinischen Histologie des menschlichen Knochenmarkes. 2. Mitteilung: Ein neues Verfahren zur histologischen Präparation von Biopsien aus Knochenmark und Knochen. Blut *14*: 30–46 (1966).

7   Lillie, R.D.; Fullmer, H.M.: Histopathologic technique and practical histochemistry, pp. 534–535 (McGraw-Hill, New York 1976).

8   De Jong, A.S.H.; Hak, T.J.; Van Duyn, P.; Daems, W.T.: A new dynamic model system for the study of capture reactions for diffusible compounds in cytochemistry. II. Effect of the composition of the incubation medium on the trapping of phosphate ions in acid cytochemistry. Histochem. J. *11*: 145–161 (1979).

9   Schmidt, P.F.; Fromme, H.G.; Pfefferkorn, G.: LAMMA-investigations of biological and medical specimens. Scanning Electron Microsc. *2*: 623–634 (1980).

10 Davison, A.M.; Ali, H.; Walker, G.S.; Lewis, A.M.: Water supply aluminium concentration, dialysis dementia, and effect of reverse-osmosis water treatment. Lancet *ii*: 785–787 (1982).

11 Fleming, L.W.; Stewart, W.K.; Fell, G.S.; Halls, D.J.: The effect of oral aluminium therapy on plasma aluminium levels in patients with chronic renal failure in an area with low water aluminium. Clin. Nephrol. *17*: 222-227 (1982).

12 Simon, M.; Bourel, M.; Faucher, R.: Association of HLA-A3 and HLA-B14 antigens with idiopathic haemochromatosis. Gut *17*: 322–334 (1976).

13 Mayor, G.H.; Keiser, J.A.; Makdani, D.; Ku, P.K.: Aluminum absorption and distribution: effect of parathyroid hormone. Science *197*: 1187–1189 (1977).

14 Parkinson, I.S.; Ward, M.K.; D.N.S.: Dialysis encephalopathy, bone disease and anemia: the aluminium intoxication syndrome during regular haemodialysis. J. clin. Path. *34*: 1285–1294 (1981).

15 Cannate, J.B.; Briggs, J.D.; Junor, R.J.; Fell, F.S.; Beastall, G.: Effect of acute aluminium overload on calcium and parathyroid-hormone metabolism. Lancet *i*: 501–503 (1983).

16 Alfrey, A.C.; LeGendre, G.R.; Kaehny, W.D.: The dialysis encephalopathy syndrome. Possible aluminium intoxication. New Engl. J. Med. *294*: 184–188 (1976).

17 Flendrig, J.A.; Kruis, H.; Das, H.A.: Aluminium intoxication: the cause of dialysis dementia? Proc. Eur. Dial. Transplant. Ass. *13*: 355–361 (1976).

18 Arieff, A.I.; Cooper, J.D.; Armstrong, D.; Lazarowitz, V.C.: Dementia, renal failure, and brain aluminium. Ann. intern. Med. *90*: 741–747 (1979).

19 Pierides, A.M.; Ward, M.K.; Kerr, D.N.S.: Haemodialysis encephalopathy: possible role of phosphate depletion. Lancet *i*: 1234–1235 (1976).

20 Mayor, G.J.; Sprague, S.M.; Sanchez, T.V.: Determinants of tissue aluminum concentrations. Am. J. Kidney Dis. *1*: 141–145 (1981).

21 Hawkins, H.K.: Reactions of lysosomes to cell injury; in Trump, Pathology of cell membranes, pp. 251–285 (Academic Press, New York 1980).

M.E. De Broe, MD, Department of Nephrology-Hypertension, Pathology and Chemistry, University of Antwerp, Wilrijkstraat 10, B-2520 Edegem (Belgium)

Contr. Nephrol., vol. 38, pp. 47–58 (Karger, Basel 1984)

Epidemiology of Aluminium Toxicity in a 'Low Incidence' Area

R.J. Winney, J.F. Cowie, A.D. Cumming, A.I.K. Short, G.D. Smith, J.S. Robson

Medical Renal Unit, Department of Medicine and Department of Pathology, Royal Infirmary, Edinburgh, Scotland, UK

Introduction

Following the observation by *Alfrey* et al. [1] that encephalopathy in patients with chronic renal failure might result from aluminium toxicity, the evidence in favour of an aluminium toxicity syndrome, particularly in patients treated by haemodialysis, has accumulated rapidly [2–10]. The major source of aluminium in haemodialysis patients is the water used for dialysis [5], but the oral ingestion of aluminium hydroxide as a phosphate binder, while rarely being the sole cause of clinical toxicity [11], also contributes to accumulation in these patients [12–13]. While most reports of aluminium toxicity have arisen from centres with very high aluminium concentrations in the water [2, 5, 7–10, 14], it seems unlikely that this problem is confined to such areas since aluminium transfer to the patient during haemodialysis occurs at very low concentrations in the dialysis fluid [15–17].

In a survey of British dialysis centres, Edinburgh had a low incidence of both encephalopathy and fracturing osteodystrophy [14]. However, following the development of encephalopathy in a home dialysis patient in 1977 an analysis of water supplies revealed considerable variation in water aluminium, although the levels were much lower than in areas with a high incidence of clinical toxicity. As a result we began a longitudinal study of plasma, water and dialysate aluminium in haemodialysis patients with the aim of defining the degree of aluminium accumulation in our patients and relating this to water and dialysis fluid aluminium as well as to possible clinical sequelae.

Patients and Methods

87 patients treated by intermittent haemodialysis were studied. At the start of the study there was no water treatment in the 37 patients treated by hospital haemodialysis and in the remainder, who were treated by home haemodialysis, the water was softened.

After an initial period of monitoring and, as a result of the initial findings, reverse osmosis water treatment was introduced if needed to maintain the dialysate aluminium <1 μmol/l. Following this the patients could be divided into three groups. In the 37 patients in group 1 on hospital haemodialysis (age 45.4 ± 11.6 years) water treatment was changed from no treatment to reverse osmosis. In the 27 patients in group 2 on home haemodialysis (age 47.4 ± 12.2 years) water treatment was changed from softening to reverse osmosis. In the 23 patients in group 3 on home haemodialysis (age 46.2 ± 10.7 years) water was treated by softening throughout the duration of the study.

Haemodialysis was conducted using a proportionating system with dialysate flow of 500 ml/min and either Cordis Dow 1.3 m^2, Asahi AM.10 1.1 m^2 or Gambro Lundia 1.1 m^2 dialysers. Patients treated by the Redy system were excluded from the study. Patients on hospital haemodialysis were treated for 5−7 h twice weekly and on home haemodialysis for 4−5 h three times weekly. All patients were prescribed aluminium-containing phosphate binders if indicated to maintain the plasma phosphate <2 mmol/l.

Untreated water and dialysate aluminium were measured monthly. In patients on hospital treatment plasma aluminium was measured monthly while in home patients estimations were performed at outpatient visits (one to three monthly).

Aluminium was analysed in duplicate samples of water, dialysis fluid and plasma by atomic absorption spectrophotometry using the Perkin Elmer 127 spectrophotometer with HGA carbon furnace [18]. The method was modified for dialysis fluid and plasma by using a continuous ramp time between 120 and 1,400°C and a total time between these temperatures of 18 s. No significant difference was found in aluminium analysis using standards with acidified (^{m}/500 nitric acid) water compared with acidified saline standards. Thus any signal suppression by sodium was slight and statistically insignificant. Similarly no significant difference was found when aluminium was analysed using plasma or serum.

In our laboratory for 29 normal people the plasma aluminium was 0.2 ± 0.07 μmol/l. In 15 patients with chronic renal failure who were not on dialysis and not treated with aluminium-containing phosphate binders the plasma aluminium was 0.47 ± 0.39 μmol/l; in a further group of 30 patients with chronic renal failure also not on dialysis but treated with aluminium-containing phosphate binders the plasma aluminium was 1.32 ± 0.7 μmol/l.

For each patient the mean water, dialysate and plasma aluminium during each method of water treatment was calculated to give an index of overall exposure. These results were then used to calculate the mean values for each group. Values in tables and text are expressed as the mean ± 1 SD.

Results

Before Introduction of Reverse Osmosis
There was marked variation in water aluminium in groups 1 and 2 with levels fluctuating from one week to another (table I.) Exposure to

Table I. Results of aluminium monitoring in haemodialysis patients before and after change to reverse osmosis (RO) water treatment

Group	Number of patients	Total duration haemodialysis months	Water treatment	Duration of observation months	Mean water aluminium μmol/l
1	37	44.2 ± 5.5	none	3.6 ± 0.9	5.6 ± 1.99
			RO	19.2 ± 10.2	–
2	27	89.3 ± 33.1	softening	12.4 ± 6.3	2.1 ± 1.5
			RO	23.3 ± 7.8	2.6 ± 1.9
3	23	71 ± 25.2	softening	36.3 ± 9.3	0.7 ± 0.2

Group	Number of patients	Mean dialysate aluminium μmol/l	Mean plasma aluminium μmol/l	Clinical toxicity (number of patients)
1	37	2.3 ± 1.5	8.2 ± 4.6	9
		0.4 ± 0.1	4.9 ± 2.8	
2	27	1.1 ± 0.7	6.4 ± 3.1	7
		0.6 ± 0.2	5.3 ± 0.4	
3	23	0.6 ± 0.2	3.9 ± 1.2	0

aluminium within each group was reflected equally by either water, dialysate or plasma aluminium which were all highest in group 1 with no water treatment, intermediate in group 2 and lowest in group 3 (table I). The incidence of clinical toxicity was also related to the degree of exposure to aluminium as assessed by either water, dialysate or plasma aluminium (table I). The plasma aluminium in group 3 was significantly lower than that in group 1 ($p < 0.001$) despite the significantly longer duration of dialysis than patients in group 1 ($p < 0.001$). For the 50 patients treated by water softening there was a significant correlation between plasma and dialysate aluminium (fig. 1) as well as between plasma and water aluminium ($r\ 0.35$; $p < 0.02$). By contrast no correlation existed between plasma aluminium and duration of dialysis in any group. In groups 1 and 2 the plasma aluminium in patients with clinical toxicity was significantly higher than that in patients without toxicity (table II).

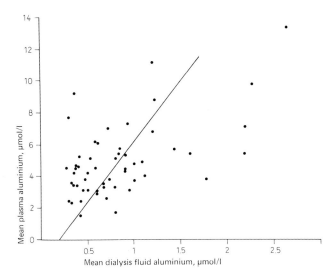

Fig. 1. Relationship between plasma and dialysis fluid aluminium in patients treated by haemodialysis using softened water. r = 0.55, p < 0.001.

The clinical severity of aluminium toxicity was in general greater in patients using untreated water than in patients using softened water (tables III, IV). A microcytic anaemia was the most common manifestation followed in frequency by fracturing osteodystrophy. Typical dialysis encephalopathy occurred in only 2 patients. The onset of a microcytic anaemia always preceded fractures or encephalopathy and was always accompanied by osteomalacia on bone biopsy (with the exception of case 4 in group 1, in whom there was no bone histology). Hyperparathyroidism was not a feature in any case, either radiologically or histologically. In patients with clinical toxicity the mean plasma aluminium was at least 8 μmol/l and, in most, much higher with the exception of cases 4–7 in group 2. These patients differed from the others both in the clinical manifestations and also in the fact that the dialysate aluminium was not documented as being consistently above 1 μmol/l. They had all been on dialysis for some years during which time they had been treated with oral aluminium hydroxide. Case 4 in group 2 did not demonstrate a fall in haemoglobin or microcytosis but had typical fracturing osteomalacia. Cases 5–7 in group 2 also did not show a fall in haemoglobin although the red cells were microcytic. They all had histological osteomalacia and, although there were no clinical

Table II. Comparison of plasma aluminium in patients with and without evidence of clinical toxicity

	Number	Plasma aluminium	
		μmol/l ± 1 SD	
Haemodialysis with no water treatment			
Patients with clinical toxicity	9	14.2 ± 3.49	p < 0.001
Patients without clinical toxicity	28	6.3 ± 3.01	
Haemodialysis using softened water			
Patients with clinical toxicity	7	9.3 ± 2.92	p < 0.001
Patients without clinical toxicity	20	5.4 ± 2.49	
No significant difference in age or duration of haemodialysis			

or electroencephalographic features typical of dialysis encephalopathy, they developed a change in well-being and personality characterised by apathy and a flat affect.

After the Introduction of Reverse Osmosis

This was associated with a significant reduction in both dialysate and plasma aluminium in groups 1 and 2 with the dialysate aluminium being maintained < 1 μmol/l (table I). The plasma aluminium fell with the reverse osmosis in all but 3 patients in whom the levels rose − in 2 cases this was unexplained and in the third case was related to the excessive ingestion of aluminium hydroxide. In patients in group 3 in whom water treatment was not altered the mean plasma aluminium at the start of the study (3.22 ± 1.51 μmol/l) had risen slightly, but significantly, to 4.2 ± 1.88 μmol/l by 30 months. With reverse osmosis water treatment there was no longer a significant correlation between plasma and dialysate aluminium. In groups 1 and 2 the mean plasma aluminium during reverse osmosis treatment was significantly correlated with the mean plasma aluminium before the introduction of reverse osmosis (r 0.72; $p < 0.001$).

Where microcytic anaemia and subclinical osteomalacia were the only clinical problems the microcytosis resolved, anaemia improved and there was no progression of bone disease (tables III, IV). Similarly, in patients

Table III. Details of clinical toxicity in haemodialysis patients using untreated water and outcome with reverse osmosis water treatment

Patient No.	Sex	Age years	Duration haemodialysis months	Microcytic anaemia	Osteo-malacia	Encephalo-pathy	Mean plasma aluminium, µmol/l		Outcome
							before RO	after RO	
1	M	63	10	+	H	−	18.4	5.5	well
2	F	18	12	+	H	−	13.9	4.6	well
3	F	59	40	+	H	−	14	4.8	well
4	F	54	13	+	?	−	11.4	6.4	well
5	F	39	30	+	C	−	10	8.3	dead
6	M	56	43	+	C	−	14.1	6.5	dead
7	M	29	34	+	C	−	13	5.3	well
8	F	64	11	+	C	+	12.4	7.3	dead
9	F	48	59	+	H	+	21.3	17.1	dead

The symbols H and C signify histological and fracturing osteomalacia, respectively. ? indicates there was no bone biopsy. The symbol + indicates present; − indicates absent.

Table IV. Details of clinical toxicity in haemodialysis patients using softened water and outcome with reverse osmosis water treatment

Patient No.	Sex	Age years	Duration haemodia- lysis months	Microcytic anaemia	Osteo- malacia	Encephalo- pathy	Mean plasma aluminium, μmol/l before RO	after RO	Outcome
1	F	59	15	+	H	–	8.1	6.3	well
2	F	42	28	+	H	–	13.4	3.4	well
3	M	24	34	+	C	–	12.8	6.3	well
4	M	47	78	–	C	–	5.1	5	well
5	M	53	45	microcytic	H	*	8.9	6.4	dead
6	M	50	64	microcytic	H	*	9.2	8.6	dead
7	M	59	81	microcytic	H	*	7.7	7.8	dead

Patients indicated * developed personality change (see text).

with microcytic anaemia and fracturing osteodystrophy the anaemia resolved and fractures healed, but 2 patients died, one as a result of sudden unexplained death and the other of neurological sequelae after a cardiac arrest. Both patients with encephalopathy died of this complication despite the fact that bone disease was arrested and despite transient improvement in neurological features in one. Similarly the 3 patients in group 2 with personality change died as a consequence of this despite the fact that bone disease did not progress. The clinical response to reverse osmosis could not be predicted from the degree of fall in plasma aluminium and improvement in complications occurred despite the fact that the plasma aluminium remained markedly elevated, although in most not in the range associated with toxicity.

Since the introduction of our policy to maintain the dialysate aluminium < 1 μmol/l we have seen no new cases with microcytic anaemia or encephalopathy and only 1 new case of fracturing osteodystrophy which was associated with excessive ingestion of aluminium hydroxide.

Influence of Aluminium Hydroxide Dosage on Plasma Aluminium

The majority of patients in group 3, in whom the dialysate aluminium had been maintained below 1 μmol/l throughout the period of observation, had been treated with oral aluminium hydroxide for some years. Despite this toxic concentrations of aluminium were not seen and there were no cases of clinical toxicity.

Following the introduction of reverse osmosis we examined the relationship between Alu-Cap® (Riker) dosage and plasma aluminium in two groups of patients. In one group in whom the dialysate aluminium had exceeded 1 μmol/l at least once in the previous 6 months as a result of malfunction of the reverse osmosis unit no correlation existed (r 0.12; p NS). By contrast, in the other group, in whom dialysate aluminium had been consistently below 1 μmol/l over the previous 6 months there was a significant correlation (fig. 2); in this group concentrations of plasma aluminium in the range associated with clinical toxicity were only seen with a daily intake of Alu-Cap in excess of 6 daily.

Discussion

This study appears to have detected a developing epidemic of aluminium toxicity in an area which had previously been recognised to have a

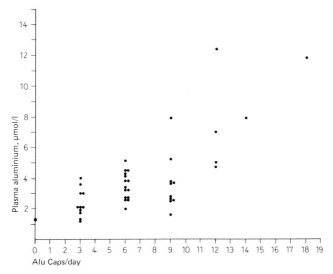

Fig. 2. Relationship of plasma aluminium to Alu-Cap dosage in haemodialysis patients: dialysate aluminium below 1 μmol/l for previous 6 months. r = 0.7, p < 0.001.

low incidence of encephalopathy and fracturing osteodystrophy. This occurred despite the fact that the aluminium content of the water supply to our patients was in general much lower than in most previous reports of aluminium toxicity [2, 5, 8–10]. However, we have observed marked fluctuation in water aluminium with occasional high peaks. Thus the finding of a low residual aluminium in a particular water supply on an isolated sample does not mean that the supply is or will continue to be safe for haemodialysis. Water softening has been shown to be an ineffective means of aluminium removal when concentrations in the water are very high [5, 10]. While at the lower levels in our area water softeners may have afforded some degree of protection they were unreliable and, occasionally, dangerous, giving the impression that they acted as a filter for aluminium with the intermittent discharge of aluminium in much higher concentrations than in the pretreatment water.

While many studies have demonstrated a close relationship between water aluminium and the incidence of clinical complications [7, 9, 14], it is the dialysis fluid aluminium concentration which determines the rate of transfer of aluminium during dialysis [19]. We have shown that the dialysis fluid aluminium is reflected both in the plasma concentration and the incidence of complications, clinical toxicity being confined to the groups in whom the dialysate aluminium was maintained above 1 μmol/l. Furthermore, a reduction in dialysate aluminium below 1 μmol/l enabled recovery of some complications and there have subsequently been no new clinical problems resulting from aluminium accumulation from dialysis fluid. This would suggest that the previously recommended safe level of aluminium in water of 2 μmol/l [2, 14] is too high and that the safe level is below 1 μmol/l, and, probably, around 0.5 μmol/l. The 'ideal' dialysis fluid aluminium concentration is one which prevents transfer of aluminium to the patient during haemodialysis and enables removal of aluminium accumulated from oral aluminium hydroxide. Recent studies would suggest that this is lower than our 'safe' concentration [15–17]. However, achieving the ideal may involve the use of complex and expensive equipment and it remains to be seen whether this is necessary to prevent clinical problems.

We have also found that the plasma aluminium is a sensitive index of the prevailing dialysate aluminium and gives a good guide to the risk of toxicity. On the basis of our experience a plasma aluminium consistently in excess of 8 μmol/l is associated with a high risk of clinical complications. While, as with others [5, 9], we found overlap in plasma aluminium in cases with toxicity compared to those without complications, this is perhaps not surprising since duration of exposure may also be important in determining the development of complications. Following removal from exposure to aluminium we have found that the plasma aluminium falls only slowly. Our experience suggests that the prevailing plasma aluminium reflects not only present but previous exposure to aluminium.

The manifestations of aluminium toxicity in our patients contrast with those in most previous studies [2, 5, 9, 10, 14]. Thus microcytic anaemia and osteomalacia, often subclinical, were the predominant findings while typical encephalopathy was uncommon. We suspect that the clinical manifestations of aluminium toxicity may vary with the degree and duration of exposure to aluminium, and this impression is supported by the findings of *Davison* et al. [2]. Thus in an area with very high aluminium levels in the water the predominant complications will be encephalopathy and fracturing osteodystrophy while at lower levels, such as in our area, the clinical syndromes will be different. Our limited experience with encephalopathy is similar to that of others, this complication tending to progress or only partially recover despite removal from exposure to aluminium [5]. By contrast, anaemia and fracturing osteodystrophy showed a good response to removal from exposure, suggesting that early detection is important if recovery is to occur. The development of microcytic anaemia in our experience is a useful early guide to aluminium toxicity since its onset appeared to precede other complications. However, despite recovery of anaemia and bone disease, 2 of our patients died suddenly tending to confirm the suggestion that aluminium may be cardiotoxic [20].

In haemodialysis patients the main risk factor for aluminium toxicity is a high aluminium concentration in the dialysis fluid. While the oral ingestion of aluminium hydroxide contributes to aluminium accumulation, toxicity from this source alone appears to be uncommon [11–13]. Only when the dialysate aluminium was maintained consistently below 1 μmol/l could we identify a significant relationship between aluminium hydroxide intake and plasma aluminium. Since plasma aluminium concentrations in the toxicity range were found with a daily intake in excess of 6 Alu-Cap (equivalent to approximately 30 ml aluminium hydroxide gel), it would seem prudent to restrict the intake of these preparations. Our experience supports the suggestion that, while toxicity as a result of aluminium hydroxide is uncommon, it does occasionally occur. In 4 of our patients we suspect that complications resulted from a combination of a slightly high dialysate aluminium and the ingestion of aluminium hydroxide for some years. Furthermore, in 3 of the patients the clinical syndrome was different to the normal pattern and included a combination of subclinical osteomalacia and vague neurological disturbance. The lower plasma aluminium concentrations in these patients compared to other patients with expected complications further support our impression that low-grade exposure to aluminium over some years may produce a different syndrome to that associated with acute exposure to high levels of aluminium in dialysis fluid.

This study illustrates the value of monitoring dialysis fluid and plasma aluminium in detecting aluminium toxicity in haemodialysis patients. Since aluminium accumulation may occur either from dialysis fluid or aluminium hydroxide we would suggest that regular monitoring of both plasma and dialysis fluid aluminium is needed to identify patients at risk of toxicity as well as the source of aluminium. With such measures the distressing syndrome of aluminium toxicity may now be able to be prevented.

References

1   Alfrey, A.; Le Gendre, G.; Kaehny, W.: The dialysis encephalopathy syndrome: possible aluminium intoxication. New Engl. J. Med. *294*: 184–188 (1976).

2   Davison, A.; Walker, G.; Oli, H.; Levins, A.: Water supply aluminium concentrations, dialysis dementia and effect of reverse-osmosis water treatment. Lancet *ii*: 785–787 (1982).

3 O'Hare, J.; Murnagham, D.: Reversal of aluminium-induced haemodialysis anaemia by a low-aluminium dialysate. New Engl. J. Med. *306*: 654–656 (1982).

4 McDermott, J.; Smith, A.; Ward, M.; Parkinson, I.; Kerr, D.: Brain-aluminium concentrations in dialysis encephalopathy. Lancet *i*: 901–904 (1978).

5 Parkinson, I.; Ward, M.; Kerr, D.: Dialysis encephalopathy, bone disease and anaemia: the aluminium intoxication syndrome during regular haemodialysis. J. clin. Path. *34*: 1285–1294 (1981).

6 Short, A.; Winney, R.; Robson, J.: Reversible microcytic hypochromic anaemia in dialysis patients due to aluminium intoxication. Proc. Eur. Dial. Transplant Ass. *17*: 226–233 (1980).

7 Report from the Registration Committee of the European Dialysis and Transplant Association: Dialysis dementia in Europe. Lancet *ii*: 190–192 (1980).

8 Ward, M.; Feest, T.; Ellis, H.; Parkinson, I.; Kerr, D.: Osteomalacic osteodystrophy: evidence for a water-borne aetiological agent, probably aluminium. Lancet *i*: 841–845 (1978).

9 Elliot, H.; Dryburgh, F.; Fell, G.; Sabet, S.; Macdougall, A.: Aluminium toxicity during regular haemodialysis. Br. med. J. *i*: 1101–1103 (1978).

10 Platts, M.; Goode, G.; Hislop, J.: Composition of the domestic water supply and the incidence of fractures and encephalopathy in patients on home dialysis. Br. med. J. *ii*: 657–660 (1977).

11 Masselot, J.; Adhemar, J.; Jaudon, M.; Klunknecht, D.; Galli, A.: Reversible dialysis encephalopathy: role for aluminium-containing gels. Lancet *ii*: 1386–1387 (1978).

12 Fleming, L.; Stewart, W.; Fell, G.; Halls, D.: The effect of oral aluminium therapy on plasma aluminium levels in patients with chronic renal failure in an area with a low water aluminium. Clin. Nephrol. *17*: 222–227 (1982).

13 Marsden, S.; Parkinson, I.; Ward, M.; Ellis, H.; Kerr, D.: Evidence for aluminium accumulation in renal failure. Proc. Eur. Dial. Transplant Ass. *16*: 588–596 (1979).

14 Parkinson, I.; Feest, T.; Ward, M.; Fawcett, R.; Kerr, D.: Fracturing dialysis osteodystrophy and dialysis encephalopathy: an epidemiological survey. Lancet *i*: 406–408 (1979).

15 Graf, H.; Stummvoll, H.; Meisinger, V.: Dialysate aluminium concentration and aluminium transfer during haemodialysis. Lancet *i*: 46–47 (1982).

16 Hodge, K.; Day, J.; O'Hara, M.; Ackrill, P.; Ralston, A.: Critical concentrations of aluminium in water used for dialysis. Lancet *ii*: 802–803 (1981).

17 Graf, H.; Stummvoll, H.; Meisinger, V.; Kovarik, J.; Wolf, A.; Pingera, W.: Aluminium removal by haemodialysis. Kidney int. *19*: 587–592 (1981).

18 Gardiner, P.; Ottoway, J.; Fell, G.; Halls, D.: Determination of aluminium in blood plasma or serum by electrothermal atomic absorption spectrometry. Analytica chim. Acta *128*: 57–66 (1981).

19 Kaehny, W.; Alfrey, A.; Holman, R.; Shorr, W.: Aluminium transfer during haemodialysis. Kidney int. *12*: 361–365 (1977).

20 Elliot, H.; Macdougall, A.; Fell, G.: Aluminium toxicity syndrome. Lancet *i*: 1203 (1978).

Dr. R.J. Winney, Medical Renal Unit, Royal Infirmary, Lauriston Place, Edinburgh EH3 9YW, Scotland (UK)

Contr. Nephrol., vol. 38, pp. 59–64 (Karger, Basel 1984)

Aluminum Osteopathy

Giulia Cournot-Witmer

Laboratoire des Tissus Calcifiés (CNRS-ER 126 et Inserm U–30),
Hôpital des Enfants Malades, Paris, France

In chronic renal failure, histologically diagnosed osteomalacia occurs, before dialysis, in about 33% of patients [1]. This bone lesion, defined as a mineralization defect of the organic matrix, is characterized by increased osteoid volume, wide osteoid seams, reduced extent of the mineralization front, and reduced mineralization rate after tetracycline labelling. Clinical symptoms, i.e., bone pain, muscular weakness, and X-ray abnormalities such as Looser's zones and pathological fractures only occur in severe cases.

Main causes of osteomalacia are deficiency of vitamin D active metabolites [2] and phosphate depletion [3]. A strong association between osteomalacic lesions, severe hypocalcemia, and acidosis has recently been reported [1]. In most cases regular hemodialysis and treatment with vitamin D, its active metabolites (25-dydroxycholecalciferol and 1,25-dihydroxycholecalciferol) or derivatives (1α-hydroxycholecalciferol) heal or improve the mineralization defect [4]. However, some hemodialyzed patients develop a form of osteomalacia which does not respond to these treatments [5–8]. In these subjects plasma calcium levels are often spontaneously elevated, and the hypercalcemia induced by vitamin D metabolites may be severe. Plasma immunoreactive parathyroid hormone (iPTH) concentrations are relatively low and, on bone sections, lesions of osteitis fibrosa are absent or minimal. Osteoid tissue has a characteristic patchy distribution. Plasma alkaline phosphatase activites are not raised. Plasma phosphorus is normal or high, thus excluding phosphate depletion. The disease may be associated with a syndrome of speech disorder, myoclonus, and dementia firstly described by *Alfrey* et al. [9] as dialysis encephalopathy.

During the past few years, it has been shown that in these patients the mineralization defect as well as the neurological symptoms are due to aluminum (Al) intoxication. Concerning the bone disease, this has been shown by epidemiological, histological, and experimental studies. Epidemiological studies were mainly performed in Great Britain and clearly showed a correlation of the incidence of the osteomalacic osteodystrophy with the Al content of the water used to prepare dialysate [10–12]. Futhermore, it has been shown that Al is excreted by the kidneys [13], and that patients with renal insufficiency retain Al in their tissues, mainly in the liver, the spleen, the lungs, the brain gray matter and the skeleton [14]. In subjects with dialysis osteomalacia, the bone Al content is correlated with the severity of the osteomalacic lesions [15] and is significantly higher than the bone Al content of patients with osteitis fibrosa or mixed lesions [15]. Moreover, in the bone tissue of a group of Al-intoxicated osteomalacic patients, we were able to show, using X-ray microanalysis and ion microscopy, that within the bone tissue, Al concentrates at the mineralizing layer of osteoid, the site where, by an active cell-mediated process the bone mineral is normally first deposited [8, 16].

Viewed by the electron microscope, the Al deposits appear as separate, hexagonal structures which emit X-rays characteristic for Al and phosphorus, but not for calcium. The hydroxyapatite needles have a normal aspect [unpublished observations]. In some cases, Al could also be localized along cement lines, which separate bone layers of different ages and contain neither cells nor collagen fibers [8]. These observations were confirmed by *Boyce* et al. [17] who used X-ray microanalysis, and by *Maloney* et al. [18] and several other investigators who employed histochemical techniques (fig. 1). Furthermore, the i.p. administration of $AlCl_3$ to rats [19] induces bone lesions similar to those observed in humans, and Al loading during total parenteral nutrition may induce osteomalacia [20]. All these observations provide evidence that Al intoxication is the cause of dialysis osteomalacia. The mean source of Al is the water used to prepare dialysate, when the water is not adequately purified, but intestinal absorption from antacids may also contribute to the intoxication.

However, the mechanism of the action of Al on bone mineralization is still unknown, and the relation between Al intoxication and the status of the parathyroid glands is not clear. In the bone tissue of most Al-intoxicated osteomalacic patients marrow fibrosis is absent; no osteoclast nor plump active osteoblasts are observed, the bone surfaces look inactive. No fluorescent tetracycline single or double labels are seen, whereas in normal

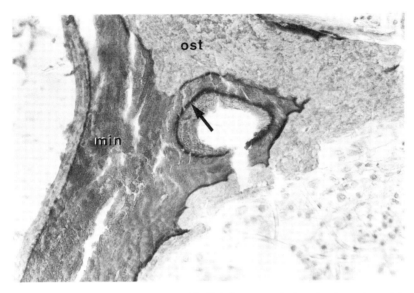

Fig. 1. Bone trabecula of a patient with dialysis osteomalacia. Aluminum (arrow) is clearly concentrated between osteoid tissue (ost) and mineralized matrix (min). Aluminon. × 235.

bone these labels are fixed at the sites of mineral deposition and allow the measurement of the rate of matrix formation and mineralization. However, some Al-intoxicated patients have severe osteitis fibrosa and minor mineralization defects [8]. In such patients, we have observed [unpublished data] that Al deposits are not only found in the bone matrix but also within the cells, i.e. in the mitochondria of the osteoblasts, cells which synthetize osteoid tissue and regulate mineralization. These observations suggest that secondary hyperparathyroidism, by increasing bone turnover, stimulates the uptake of Al by the osteoblasts and its release into the organic matrix. Indeed in rats, administration of PTH increases the bone Al concentration [21]. Furthermore, in hemodialyzed patients, an inverse correlation has been reported between serum iPTH concentration and the severity of Al intoxication, evaluated by the bone Al content [7]. Significantly higher serum Al and calcium values were observed in a group of hemodialyzed patients with lower serum iPTH concentrations, compared with those of a control group with higher iPTH concentrations [22]. Subjects with dialysis osteomalacia have an almost normal plasma iPTH and, moreover, in these patients low calcium dialysate does not increase the iPTH concentration, in contrast to what occurs in control patients [23]. In addition, *Cann* et al. [24] reported that parathyroid glands preferentially accumulate Al.

All these observations taken together suggest that: (1) the presence of Al within the mitochondria of the osteoblasts may gradually intoxicate the cell, being one of the factors inducing the mineralization defect; (2) Al has a direct toxic action on parathyroid glands. This action may be at the origin of the low iPTH plasma levels observed in the osteomalacic patients and may contribute to the low bone cellular activity and turnover observed in these patients.

In conclusion, Al osteopathy is a form of osteomalacia induced by Al intoxication (dialysis osteomalacia, low-turnover osteomalacia) occurring mainly in hemodialyzed patients. In these osteomalacic patients severe secondary hyperparathyroidism is lacking. The bone lesions do not respond to vitamin D treatment. This treatment may induce severe hypercalcemia. Al osteopathy is diagnosed on histological sections by the presence of Al along the mineralization front, by the patchy distribution of osteoid, and the almost complete absence of active bone cells and marrow fibrosis.

Dialysis osteomalacia may be prevented by adequate water treatment with reverse osmosis or deionization and, in patients receiving large doses of antacids, by avoiding persistent hyperaluminemia. Some recent data suggests the effectiveness of an Al-chelating agent, i.e. desferrioxamine, in improving these bone lesions [25, 26].

References

1   Mora Palma, F.J.; Lorenzo Sellares, V.; Ellis, H.A.; Ward, M.K.; Kerr, D.N.S.: Osteomalacia in chronic renal failure before dialysis. Proc. Eur. Dial. Transplant Ass. *19*: 188–194 (1982).

2   Stanbury, S.W.: The role of vitamin D in renal bone disease. Clin. Endocrinol. 7: suppl., pp. 25S–30S (1977).

3   Baker, L.R.I.; Ackrill, P.; Cattell, W.R.; Stamp, T.C.B.; Watson, L.: Iatrogenic osteomalacia and myopathy due to phosphate depletion. Br. med. J. *iii*: 150–152 (1974).

4   Witmer, G.; Margolis, A.; Fontaine, O.; Fritsch, J.; Lenoir, G.; Broyer, M.; Balsan, S.: Effects of 25-hydroxycholecalciferol on bone lesions of children with terminal renal failure. Kidney int. *10*: 395–408 (1976).

5   Ellis, H.A.; Pierides, A.M.; Feest, T.G.; Ward, M.K.; Kerr, D.N.S.: Histopathology of renal osteodystrophy with particular reference to the effects of 1α-hydroxyvitamin D₃ in patients treated by long-term haemodialysis. Clin. Endocrinol. 7: suppl., pp. 31S–38S (1977).

6 Coburn, J.W.; Brickman, A.S.; Sherrard, D.J.; Singer, F.R.; Wong, E.G.C.; Baylink, D.J.; Norman, A.W.: Use of 1,25(OH)$_2$-vitamin D$_3$ to separate 'types' of renal osteodystrophy. Proc. Eur. Dial. Transplant Ass. *14*: 442−450 (1977).

7 Hodsman, A.B.; Sherrard, D.J.; Wong, G.C.; Brickman, A.S.; Lee, B.N.; Alfrey, A.C.; Singer, F.R.; Norman, A.W.; Coburn, J.W.: Vitamin-D-resistant osteomalacia in hemodialysis patients lacking secondary haperparathyroidism. Ann. intern. Med. *94*: 629−637 (1981).

8 Cournot-Witmer, G.; Zingraff, J.; Plachot, J.J.; Escaig, F.; Lefevre, R.; Boumati, P.; Bourdeau, A.; Garabédian, M.; Galle, P.; Bourdon, R.; Drüeke, T.; Balsan, S.: Aluminium localization in bone from hemodialyzed patients: Relationship to matrix mineralization. Kidney int. *80*: 375−385 (1981).

9 Alfrey, A.C., Le Gendre, G.R.; Kaehny, W.D.: The dialysis encephalopathy syndrome: possible aluminium intoxication. New Engl. J. Med. *294*: 184−188 (1976).

10 Platts, M.M.; Goode, G.C.; Hislop, J.S.: Composition of the domestic water supply and the incidence of fractures and encephalopathy in patients on home dialysis. Br. med. J. *ii*: 657−660 (1977).

11 Ward, M.K.; Feest, T.G.; Ellis, H.A.; Parkinson, I.S.; Kerr, D.N.S.: Osteomalacic dialysis osteodystrophy: evidence for a water-borne aetiological agent, probably aluminium. Lancet *i*: 841−845 (1978).

12 Parkinson, I.S.; Ward, M.K.; Feest, T.G.; Fawcett, R.W.P.; Kerr, D.N.S.: Fracturing dialysis osteodystrophy and dialysis encephalopathy. Lancet *i*: 406−409 (1979).

13 Kovalchik, M.T.; Kaehny, W.D.; Hegg, A.P.; Jackson, J.T.; Alfrey, A.C.: Aluminium kinetics during hemodialysis. J. Lab. clin. Med. *92*: 712−720 (1978).

14 Alfrey, A.C.; Hegg, A.; Craswell, P.: Metabolism and toxicity of aluminium in renal failure. Am. J. clin. Nutr. *33*: 1509−1516 (1980).

15 Hodsman, A.B.; Sherrad, D.J.; Alfrey, A.C.; Ott, S.; Brickman, A.S.; Miller, N.L.; Maloney, N.A.; Coburn, J.W.: Bone aluminium and histomorphometric features of renal osteodystrophy. J. clin. Endocr. Metab. *54*: 539−546 (1982).

16 Lefevre, R.; Cournot-Witmer, G.; Galle, P.: Electron microprobe analysis and analytical ion microscopy of normal and pathological bone (dialysis osteomalacia). Scann. Electron Microsc. *3*: 106−107 (1980).

17 Boyce, B.F.; Elder, H.Y.; Fell, G.S.; Nicholson, W.A.P.; Smith, G.D.; Dempster, D.W.; Gray, C.C.; Boyle, I.T.: Quantitation and localization of aluminium in human cancellous bone in renal osteodystrophy. Scann. Electron. Microsc. *3*: 329−337 (1981).

18 Maloney, N.A.; Ott, S.M.; Alfrey, A.C.; Miller, N.L.; Coburn, J.W.: Histological quantitation of aluminium in iliac bone from patients with renal failure. J. Lab. clin. Med. *99*: 206−216 (1982).

19 Ellis, H.A.; McCarthy, J.H.; Herrington, J.: Bone aluminium in hemodialyzed patients and in rats injected with aluminium chloride: relationship to impaired bone mineralization. J. clin. Path. *32*: 832−844 (1979).

20 Klein, G.L.; Alfrey, A.C.; Miller, N.L.; Sherrard, D.J.; Hazlet, T.K.; Ament, M.E.; Coburn, J.W.: Aluminium loading during total parenteral nutrition. Am. J. clin. Nutr. *35*: 1425−1429 (1982).

21 Mayor, G.H.; Keiser, J.A.; Makdani, D.; Ku, P.K.: Aluminium absorption and distribution: effect of parathyroid hormone. Science *197*: 1187−1189 (1977).

22 Cannata, J.B.; Briggs, J.D.; Junor, B.J.R.; Beastall, G.; Fell, G.S.: The influence of

aluminium on parathyroid hormone levels in haemodialysis patients. Proc. Eur. Dial. Transplant Ass. *19*: 244–247 (1982).

23   Kraut, J.A.; Shinaberger, F.R.; Singer, D.J.; Sherrard, J.; Hodsman, A.B.; Miller, J.H.; Kurokawa, K.; Coburn, J.W.: Reduced parathyroid response to acute hypocalcemia in dialysis osteomalacia. Clin. Res. *29*: 102A (1981).

24   Cann, C.E.; Prussin, S.G.; Gordan, G.S.: Aluminium uptake by the parathyroid glands. J. clin. Endocr. Metab. *49*: 543–545 (1979).

25   Ackrill, P.; Day, J.P.; Garstang, F.M.; Hodge, K.C.; Metcalfe, P.J.; Benzo, Z.; Hill, K.; Ralston, A.J.; Ball, J.; Denton, J.: Treatment of fracturing renal osteodystrophy by desferrioxamine. Proc. Eur. Dial. Transplant Ass. *19*: 203–207 (1982).

26   Ihle, B.U.; Buchanan, M.R.C.; Stevens, B.; Becker, G.J.; Kincaid-Smith, P.: The efficacy of various treatment modalities on aluminium associated bone disease. Proc. Eur. Dial. Transplant Ass. *19*: 195–202 (1982).

G. Cournot-Witmer, MD, Laboratoire des Tissus Calcifiés (CNRS-ER 126 et Inserm U-30), Hôpital des Enfants Malades, F-75015 Paris (France)

Contr. Nephrol., vol. 38, pp. 65–77 (Karger, Basel 1984)

Therapy of Aluminum Overload (I)

A.M. Pierides, M. Pierce Myli

Division of Nephrology and Department of Medical Pathology, Mayo Clinic, Rochester, Minn., USA

Introduction

Patients with renal failure have a reduced capacity to excrete aluminum in the urine, and any excess aluminum that enters the body tends to accumulate in blood and other body tissues [1–4]. Dietary aluminum and aluminum released while cooking in aluminum utensils [5] are potential sources of aluminum, but the most significant source for nondialyzed azotemic patients is the aluminum contained in phosphate binders prescribed to azotemic patients for the prevention and treatment of hyperphosphatemia [6–9]. Prolonged ingestion of large quantities of these gels has led to the development of aluminum encephalopathy and osteomalacia in azotemic patients who have never been on hemodialysis [10–12]. During repetitive hemodialysis oral aluminum-containing phosphate binders remain a problem, but a bigger danger is the use of aluminum contaminated dialysate solutions [1, 2, 4, 13, 14]. Dialysate solutions with aluminum concentrations over 100 µg/l have been responsible for the epidemics of aluminum encephalopathy and osteomalacia in Ottawa [15], Denver [1, 16], Newcastle Upon Tyne [4, 17], Chicago [18], Plymouth [19], and Columbia S.C. [20]. Aluminum contaminated peritoneal solutions have also led to aluminum overload in CAPD patients [21, 22], and dialysis sorbents containing aluminum such as the Redy cartridge have been incriminated in the development of aluminum osteomalacia and encephalopathy [23, 24].

While the clinical syndromes of aluminum osteomalacia and encephalopathy are now well known, no effective and reliable method for removing aluminum was available until *Ackrill* et al. [25] reported on the beneficial effect of long-term deferoxamine in a patient with aluminum en-

Table I. Clinical characteristics and bone histomorphometry in 5 hemodialysis patients prior to treatment with deferoxamine

Patient No.	Age	Sex	Months on hemodialysis	Symptoms of encephalopathy	Bone histology		
					osteomalacia	osteitis fibrosa grade 0−5	aluminum stain
1	60	M	108	yes	yes	0	positive
2	29	M	78	no	yes	0.5	positive
3	42	F	84	no	yes	1.0	positive
4[1]	58	M	35	yes	yes	1.0	positive
5	59	M	121	yes	yes	1.0	positive

[1] Patient dialyzed with the Redy sorbent cartridge.

cephalopathy. Their observation has since been confirmed [26−29]. This report describes our experience in treating 5 aluminum-overloaded hemodialysis patients with long-term deferoxamine. The report also describes our experience in treating and preventing aluminum overload with water purification and also the role of successful renal transplantation in the management of aluminum osteomalacia and encephalopathy.

Long-Term Deferoxamine Therapy

Since March 1981, 5 patients with histologically confirmed aluminum overload and osteomalacia have been treated with long-term deferoxamine (table I). 3 patients had symptoms of aluminum encephalopathy. 1 patient dialyzed with the Redy sorbent cartridge. The mean period on hemodialysis was 85 months (35−121). At the beginning of the study all patients received a transiliac bone biopsy, and staining for aluminum by means of the aurine tricarboxylic acid technique was strongly positive in all patients (fig. 1). During the first treatment 1 g of deferoxamine dissolved in 200 ml of 0.9% saline was administered slowly over a 2-hour period. This was done in order to detect any allergic reactions to deferoxamine. On the next hemodialysis session 4 g of deferoxamine dissolved in 200 ml of 0.9% saline were administered intravenously during the first half hour of hemodialysis. This treatment was repeated with every third dialysis. Every 4−6 weeks the blood aluminum clearance was measured 2 h after the ad-

Table II. Aluminum clearance during hemodialysis with a CF1511 filter and 4 g Desferal

Patient	QB, ml/min	Simultaneous plasma aluminum concentration, µg/l		Simultaneous dialysate aluminum concentration, µg/l		Clearance, ml/min
		arterial (predialyzer)	venous (postdialyzer)	(predialyzer)	(postdialyzer)	
1	200	115	99	18	26	27.8
	207	143	109	8	26	49.2
2	203	328	260	<2.5	31	42.1
	200	281	234	<2.5	4	32.0
3	200	301	220	<2.5	9	53.8
4	205	310	268	<2.5	10	27.7
5	195	225	190	<2.5	9.6	30.3

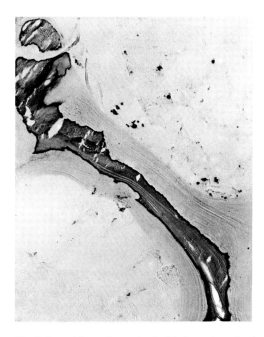

Fig. 1. 3 µm thin section stained with the aurine tricarboxylic acid technique to illustrate severe osteomalacia and aluminum deposition. Mineralized bone in the center of the trabeculum appears dark. Osteoid is pale on the outside. The aluminum is deposited in a linear fashion along the interphase of mineralized bone and osteoid. × 160.

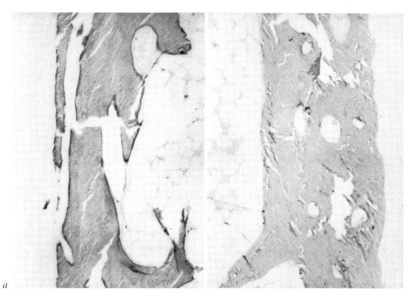

Fig. 2a, b. Sections stained for aluminum before and after 1 year of deferoxamine. The pink aluminum stain has largely disappeared after treatment with 4 g of Desferal weekly for 1 year. × 64.

ministration of deferoxamine. The blood flow 'Q_B' was determined with the bubble transit technique, and simultaneous blood and dialysate specimens were obtained pre- and postdialyzer. The formula:

$$\text{Clearance} = \frac{Q_B (C_{Bi} - C_{Bo})}{C_{Bi}} ,$$

was used to calculate the aluminum clearance. Table II summarizes the aluminum clearance in these 5 patients dialyzing with a Travenol CF1511 dialyzer. The mean aluminum clearance was 37.5 ml/min. 1 patient has completed 1 year of treatment and has undergone a post-treatment bone biopsy (fig. 2a, b). The remaining 4 patients have been treated for less than 1 year. No allergic reactions or other side effects have been observed in any of these 5 patients. Relief of skeletal and encephalopathic symptoms have been observed in the first 3 patients who have been treated for 20, 8 and 6 months, respectively. The following case histories illustrate the findings in the first 2 patients.

Table III. Plasma aluminum during long-term treatment with 4 g Desferal i.v. weekly Patient 1

		Simultaneous plasma aluminum concentrations μg/l			
		arterial (predialyzer)	venous (postdialyzer)	bone Al ppm	predialysis plasma Al
1981	Mar. 2	328	324	415	135
	May 21	127	113		
	July 15	250	242		
	Oct. 17	143	109		
1982	Feb. 19	139	109		
	June 2	103	99	159	39
		Desferal stopped June → Oct. 1982			
	Oct. 29	169	89		
	Dec. 3	86	79		

Case Histories

Patient 1 (table I). After 9 years on home hemodialysis with a dialysate solution prepared with water from reverse osmosis and deionization, this patient developed speech problems, seizures, muscle weakness, and pain in both groins and hips. The EEG was compatible with dialysis encephalopathy, and pelvic X-rays showed bilateral femoral neck Looser's zones. After a bone biopsy which confirmed the presence of aluminum osteomalacia, the patient was started in March 1981 on long-term deferoxamine. In August 1981, the patient was prescribed 25-OHD$_3$ 50 μg daily. Definite improvement in the patient's encephalopathic symptoms occurred over the next few months, and a repeat bone biopsy 1 year later showed resolution of the osteomalacia and a marked decrease in the aluminum staining on the bone biopsy (fig. 2a, b). Table III summarizes the serial aluminum data on this patient. The bone aluminum decreased from a pretreatment value of 415 to 159 ppm. The serum aluminum 2 h after deferoxamine also diminished over 15 months from 328 to 103 μg/l, and the predialysis serum aluminum fell from 135 to 39 μg/l. The fractures healed.

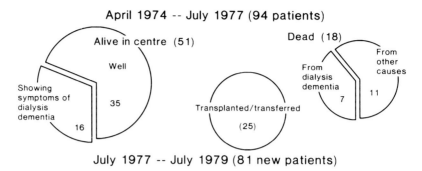

Fig. 3. Evolution of aluminum encephalopathy after water purification in Columbia S.C. (1974–1979). Following the use of aluminium-free dialysis fluid in October 1977, no new cases of dialysis dementia appeared either among the older or the new patients. 12/16 affected patients improved.

Patient 2 (table I). This 29-year-old patient had been devastated by two failed transplants in March 1976 and August 1977. As a result of significant steroid therapy he developed avascular necrosis of both hips which required total bilateral hip arthroplasties. Between 1976 and 1982 he dialyzed in a center with minimal water purification. In 1981 he began to complain of muscle weakness and pain around his ribs where several fractures developed. He was spontaneously hypercalcemic while dialyzing with a dialysate solution containing 3.25 mEq/l (6.5 mg/100 ml) of calcium, and the hypercalcemia worsened rapidly on treatment with $1,25(OH)_2D_3$. Two bone biopsies in 1980 and 1981 showed progressive osteomalacia with strong staining for aluminum. In June 1982, he began treatment with deferoxamine, 4 g each week. By February 1983, the serum aluminum, 2 h after deferoxamine, decreased from 457 to 201 µg/l. Good improvement was observed in the patient's muscle strength, and the serum calcium fell so that the patient now remains normocalcemic on treatment with 0.5 µg/l of $1,25(OH)_2D_3$ and 1.5 g of calcium carbonate daily.

Water Purification

The effect of water purification on aluminum removal and prevention of aluminum overload was studied during the epidemic of hemodialysis os-

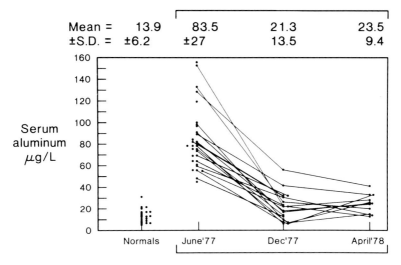

Fig. 4. Decline in serum aluminum after water purification was installed in September 1977, Columbia S.C.

teomalacia and encephalopathy in Columbia S.C. [20]. This dialysis unit opened in April, 1974, and untreated water from the Broad River was used to prepare the dialysate solution. Aluminum sulfate in variable amounts was added daily by the Columbia City Water Department. By June 1977, 7 patients had died of dialysis encephalopathy, and 16 other patients were clinically affected (fig. 3). In June 1977, the dialysate aluminum concentration was high at 140 µg/l. A water purification plant incorporating a water softener, reverse osmosis, and deionization was installed in September 1977, and the dialysate aluminum concentration fell to less than 2.5 µg/l. Figure 4 shows the progressive decline in the patients' serum aluminum concentration after the introduction of the water purification plant. Between July 1977 and July 1979, 81 new patients were accepted on the dialysis program. None of the previous or new patients developed any encephalopathic symptoms, and 12 of the 16 previously affected patients gradually improved (fig. 3). 9 months after water purification the mean hematocrit had risen significantly from a pretreatment value of 25.5 to 29.5, p < 0.001.

Successful Renal Transplantation

Beginning in 1971, a prospective study on the effect of successful renal transplantation on bone histomorphometry was undertaken at the University of Newcastle Upon Tyne [30]. At the time a large number of hemodialysis patients in that center suffered from the low turnover, normal alkaline phosphatase, osteomalacic fracture osteodystrophy, later shown to be the result of aluminum overload. Empirically, it had been observed that pathological fractures in these patients often healed after successful renal transplantation. 20 successfully transplanted patients with a serum creatinine less than 2.0 mg/100 ml 2 years after renal transplantation, received a bone biopsy on the day of the renal transplant and 1 and 2 years later. The mean % mineralization on the day of the transplant was low at 93.64. It rose to 96.13 and 97.36, 1 and 2 years later. Similarly, the mean % osteoid fell from a high pretransplant value of 1.67 to 0.81 and 0.41, 1 and 2 years later. In patients with histologically pure osteomalacia the serum total alkaline phosphatase rose spontaneously and subsequently returned to normal over the following 9–18 months [30]. The serum PTH which was low normal or undetectable in several of these osteomalacic patients rose as the aluminum osteomalacia healed (fig. 5a, b).

Discussion

Though aluminum toxicity in azotemic patients became generally recognized after 1976 [1, 2, 4, 31], clinical problems such as encephalopathy and osteomalacia with fractures had been described much earlier [15, 32, 33]. Aluminum overload is largely an iatrogenic disease, the result of our failure to recognize early enough the potential for accumulation and toxicity by trace elements such as aluminum. Prior to Ackrill's use of deferoxamine to remove aluminum, successful renal transplantation was the only other form of therapy possible [30]. Unfortunately, successful renal transplantation could not be guaranteed in every case, and a failed renal transplant often worsened the situation. Therefore, prevention of aluminum overload is of paramount importance, and it should not be possible for any azotemic patient to receive long-term treatment with hemodialysis, peritoneal dialysis or postdilution hemofiltration using aluminum contaminated dialysate solutions. Water purification with a softener, reverse osmosis and deionization should be employed in every case.

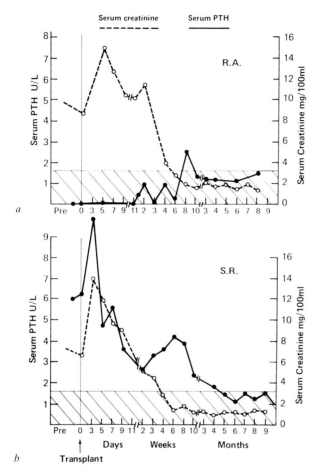

Fig. 5. Comparison of serum PTH changes after successful renal transplantation in patient R.A. (*a*) with histologically pure osteomalacia and patient S.R. (*b*) with osteitis fibrosa. The serum PTH in the patient with aluminum osteomalacia rose after renal transplantation as the osteomalacia improved, while in patient S.R. with osteitis fibrosa it gradually returned to within the normal range.

The question of oral aluminum-containing phosphate binders is a more difficult one, since these agents are generally useful, and no serious alternatives are in sight. However, prolonged consumption of these agents also leads to significant aluminum overload, and patients 1 and 5 (table I) are representative examples.

Aluminum Encephalopathy

The treatment of aluminum encephalopathy remains worrisome. Despite occasional reports of clinical improvement after cessation of oral aluminum-containing phosphate binders [34–36], water purification [13, 20], and successful renal transplantation [37, 38], this condition has a largely unfavorable prognosis and a poor long-term outcome. In general, renal transplantation often aggravates the encephalopathy, and it should be avoided especially if symptoms are severe [39]. Treatment with deferoxamine promises to be the treatment of choice in these patients, and it may also be useful prior to or after renal transplantation if this is attempted [25–27, 29].

Aluminum Osteomalacia

The clinical, radiological and histological descriptions of aluminum osteomalacia were primarily described at the University of Newcastle Upon Tyne, and this condition is often called 'Newcastle Bone Disease' [4, 8, 17, 26, 30, 32, 33]. In its early stages the disease may remain asymptomatic, but eventually bone pain, particularly affecting the ribs, feet, and pelvis develops in a large number of patients. Biochemically, the serum total alkaline phosphatase may be normal, and the total serum calcium may be normal, high normal or frankly elevated. This osteomalacia does not respond to treatment with vitamin D alone, and hypercalcemia usually develops rather promptly. Given a patient with suspected aluminum osteomalacia, a bone biopsy is always necessary to confirm the diagnosis, and the serum and dialysate aluminum concentrations should be checked. If aluminum overload with osteomalacia is confirmed, the patient should be dialyzed with an aluminum-free dialysate, and serious attempts should be made to identify a well-matched living or cadaveric renal transplant. Transplantation may be the best long-term form of therapy [30]. When successful renal transplantation is not possible, aluminum removal with long-term deferoxamine appears the treatment of choice. Long-term therapy may be required, and concurrent treatment with $1,25(OH)_2D_3$ or $25\text{-}OHD_3$ appears beneficial.

References

1   Alfrey, A.C.; LeGendre, G.R.; Kaehny, W.D.: The dialysis encephalopathy syndrome. Possible aluminum intoxication. New Engl. J. Med. *294*: 184–188 (1976).

2   Flendrig, J.A.; Kruis, H.; Das, H.A.: Aluminium intoxication: the cause of dialysis de-
    mentia? Proc. Eur. Dial. Transplant. Ass. *13*: 353–363 (1976).
3   Williams, E.D.; Elliott, H.L.; Boddy, K.; Haywood, J.K.; Henderson, I.S.; Harvey,
    I.; Kennedy, A.C.: Whole body aluminium in chronic renal failure and dialysis en-
    cephalopathy. Clin. Nephrol. *14*: 198–200 (1980).
4   McDermott, J.R.; Smith, A.I.; Ward, M.K.; Parkinson, I.S.; Kerr, D.N.S.: Brain-
    aluminium concentration in dialysis encephalopathy. Lancet *i*: 901–903 (1978).
5   Trapp, G.A.; Cannon, J.B.: Aluminum pots as a source of dietary aluminum. New
    Engl. J. Med. *304*: 172–173 (1981).
6   Clarkson, E.M.; Lukc, V.A.; Hynson, W.V.; Bailey, R.R.; Eastwood, J.B.;
    Woodhead, J.S.; Clements, V.R.; O'Riordan, J.L.H.; DeWardener, H.E.: The effect
    of aluminium hydroxide on calcium, phosphorus and aluminium balances, the serum
    parathyroid hormone concentration and the aluminium content of bone in patients with
    chronic renal failure. Clin. Sci. *43*: 519–531 (1972).
7   Boukari, M.; Rottembourg, J.; Jaudon, M.C.; Clavel, J.P.; Legrain, M.; Galli, A.: In-
    fluence de la prise prolongée de gels d'alumine sur les taux sériques d'aluminium chez
    les patients atteints d'insuffisance rénale chronique. Nouv. Presse méd. *7*: 85–88
    (1977).
8   Marsden, S.N.E.; Parkinson, I.S.; Ward, M.K.; Ellis, H.A.; Kerr, D.N.S.: Evidence
    for aluminium accumulation in renal failure. Proc. Eur. Dial. Transplant. Ass. *16*:
    588–596 (1979).
9   Fleming, L.W.; Stewart, W.K.; Fell, G.S.; Halls, D.J.: The effect of oral aluminium
    therapy on plasma aluminium levels in patients with chronic renal failure in an area with
    low water aluminium. Clin. Nephrol. *17*: 222–227 (1982).
10 Nathan, E.; Pedersen, S.E.: Dialysis encephalopathy in a non-dialysed uraemic boy
    treated with aluminium hydroxide orally. Acta paediat. scand. *69*: 793–796 (1980).
11 Etheridge, W.B.; O'Neill, W.M., Jr.: The 'dialysis encephalopathy syndrome' without
    dialysis. Clin. Nephrol. *10*: 250–252 (1978).
12 Baluarte, H.J.; Gruskin, A.B.; Hiner, L.B.; Foley, C.M.; Grover, W.D.: En-
    cephalopathy in children with chronic renal failure. Proc. Dial. Transplant. Forum *7*:
    95–97 (1977).
13 Platts, M.M.; Goode, G.C.; Hislop, J.S.: Composition of the domestic water supply
    and the incidence of fractures and encephalopathy in patients on home dialysis. Br.
    med. J. *ii*: 657–660 (1977).
14 Elliott, H.L.; Dryburgh, F.; Fell, G.S.; Sabet, S.; MacDougall, A.I.: Aluminium toxic-
    ity regular haemodialysis. Br. med. J. *i*: 1101–1103 (1978).
15 Posen, G.A.; Gray, D.G.; Jaworsky, Z.F.; Couture, R.; Rashid, A.: Comparison of
    renal osteodystrophy in patients dialyzed with de-ionized and non-deionized water.
    Trans. Am. Soc. artif. internal. Organs *18*: 405–411 (1972).
16 Alfrey, A.C.; Mishell, J.M.; Burks, J.; Contiguglia, S.; Rudolph, H.; Lewin, E.;
    Holmes, J.H.: Syndrome of dyspraxia and multifocal seizures associated with chronic
    hemodialysis. Trans. Am. Soc. artif. internal. Organs. *18*: 257–261 (1972).
17 Ward, M.K.; Ellis, H.A.; Feest, T.G.; Parkinson, I.S.; Kerr, D.N.S.; Herrington, J.;
    Goode, G.L.: Osteomalacic dialysis osteodystrophy: evidence for a water-borne
    aetiological agent, probably aluminium. Lancet *i*: 841–845 (1978).
18 Dunea, G.; Mahurkar, S.D.; Mamdani, B.; Smith, E.C.: Role of aluminum in dialysis
    dementia. Ann. intern. Med. *88*: 502–504 (1978).

19 Leather, H.M.; Lewin, I.G.; Calder, E.; Braybrooke, J.; Cox, R.R.: Effect of water deionisers on 'fracturing osteodystrophy' and dialysis encephalopathy in Plymouth. Nephron 29: 80–84 (1981).

20 Pierides, A.M.; Edwards, W.G.; Cullum, U.X.; McCall, J.T.; Ellis, H.A.: Hemodialysis encephalopathy with osteomalacic fractures and muscle weakness. Kidney int. 18: 115–124 (1980).

21 Wolf, A.; Graf, H.; Pinggera, W.F.; Stummvoll, H.K.; Meisinger, V.: Serum aluminum and continuous ambulatory peritoneal dialysis. Ann. intern. Med. 92: 130–131 (1980).

22 Sorkin, M.I.; Nolph, K.D.; Anderson, H.O.; Morris, J.S.; Kennedy, J.; Prowant, B.; Moore, H.: Aluminum mass transfer during continuous ambulatory peritoneal dialysis. Periton. Dial. Bull. 1: 91–93 (1981).

23 Mion, C.; Branger, B.; Issautier, R.; Ellis, H.A.; Rodier, M.; Shaldon, S.: Dialysis fracturing osteomalacia without hyperparathyroidism in patients treated with HCO_3 rinsed Redy cartridge. Trans. Am. Soc. artif. internal. Organs 27: 634–638 (1981).

24 Pierides, A.M.; Frohnert, P.P.: Aluminum related dialysis osteomalacia and dementia after prolonged use of the Redy cartridge. Trans. Am. Soc. artif. internal. Organs 27: 629–633 (1981).

25 Ackrill, P.; Ralston, A.J.; Day, J.P.; Hodge, K.C.: Successful removal of aluminium from patient with dialysis encephalopathy. Lancet ii: 692–693 (1980).

26 Arze, R.S.; Parkinson, I.S.; Cartlidge, N.E.F.; Britton, P.; Ward, M.K.: Reversal of aluminium dialysis encephalopathy after desferrioxamine treatment. Lancet ii: 1116 (1981).

27 Brown, D.J.; Ham, K.N.; Dawborn, J.K.; Xipell, J.M.: Treatment of dialysis osteomalacia with desferrioxamine. Lancet ii: 343–345 (1982).

28 Mudde, A.H.; Roodvoets, A.P.: Desferrioxamine and osteomalacia. Lancet ii: 608 (1982).

29 Milne, F.J.; Sharf, B.; Bell, P.D.; Meyers, A.M.: Low aluminium water, desferrioxamine, and dialysis encephalopathy. Lancet ii: 502 (1982).

30 Pierides, A.M.; Ellis, H.A.; Peart, K.M.; Simpson, W.; Uldall, P.R.; Kerr, D.N.S.: Assessment of renal osteodystrophy following renal transplantation. Proc. Eur. Dial. Transplant. Ass. 11: 481–487 (1974).

31 Ihle, B.; Buchanan, M.; Stevens, B.; Marshal, A.; Plomley, R.; d'Apice, A.; Kincaid-Smith, P.: Aluminum associated bone disease: clinicopathologic correlation. Am. J. Kidney Dis. 2: 255–263 (1982).

32 Simpson, W.; Kerr, D.N.S.; Hill, A.V.L.; Siddiqui, J.Y.: Skeletal changes in patients on regular haemodialysis. Radiology 107: 313–320 (1973).

33 Simpson, W.; Ellis, H.A.; Kerr, D.N.S.; McElroy, M.; McNay, R.A.; Peart, K.M.: Bone disease in long-term haemodialysis. The association of radiological with histological abnormalities. Br. J. Radiol. 49: 105–110 (1976).

34 Masselot, J.P.; Adhemar, J.P.; Jaudon, M.C.; Kleinknecht, D.; Galli, A.: Reversible dialysis encephalopathy: Role for aluminium-containing gels. Lancet ii: 1386–1387 (1979).

35 Poisson, M.; Mashaly, R.; Lebkiri, B.: Dialysis encephalopathy: recovery after interruption of aluminium intake. Br. med. J. ii: 1610–1611 (1978).

36 Buge, A.; Poisson, M.; Masson, S.; Bleibel, J.M.; Mashaly, R.; Jaudon, M.C.; Lafforgue, B.; Lebkiri, B.; Raymond, P.: Encéphalopathie réversible des dialysés après arrêt de l'apport d'aluminium. Nouv. Presse méd. 8: 2729–2733 (1979).

37   Sullivan, P.A.; Murnaghan, D.J.; Callaghan, N.: Dialysis dementia: recovery after transplantation. Br. med. J. *ii*: 740 (1977).
38   Mittal, V.K.; Sharma, M.J.; Toledo-Pereyra, L.H.; Baskin, S.; McNichol, L.J.: Complete recovery from dialysis dementia following kidney transplantation. Dial. Transplant. *10*: 41−42 (1981).
39   Mattern, W.D.; Krigman, M.R.; Blythe, W.B.: Failure of successful renal transplantation to reverse the dialysis-associated encephalopathy syndrome. Clin. Nephrol. 7: 275−278 (1977).

A.M. Pierides, MD, FACP, Internal Medicine and Nephrology, P.O. Box 5638, Nicosia (Cyprus)

Contr. Nephrol., vol. 38, pp. 78–80 (Karger, Basel 1984)

Therapy of Aluminium Overload (II)

P. Ackrill, J.P. Day

Department of Chemistry, Manchester University and Withington Hospital, Manchester, UK

The numerous options available for treating the variety of clinical and pathological manifestations of aluminium toxicity in patients with renal failure have been ably reviewed by Dr. *Pierides*. I will confine my remarks to methods of aluminium removal in such patients.

Clearly, all sources of continued exposure must be eliminated as the first step. This includes not only prescribed aluminium-containing oral phosphate binders, but also self-administered commercial antacids. Alternative phosphate-binding agents may be required such as magnesium hydroxide and calcium carbonate and we are currently studying the binding effects of ferric hydroxide.

Controversy continues regarding what is a safe dialysate aluminium concentration, but we have previously shown [1] that in order to achieve a negative aluminium balance during haemodialysis, the aluminium levels should be below 14 µg/l (0.5 µmol/l). To reduce dialysate aluminium levels, attention has largely been paid to removal of aluminium from the dialysate water supply. It is nevertheless equally important to consider the aluminium content of dialysate concentrate and likewise of replacement fluids during haemofiltration, plasmaphaeresis, blood transfusion, etc.

The introduction of adequate water treatment has resulted in not only elimination of new cases in a number of previously affected renal units, but also improvement in some of the affected patients. Both reduction of ingested aluminium and reduction in dialysate aluminium result in profound falls in serum aluminium concentration but how much this is due to reduction of the body burden is not certain. We and others have shown that it is possible to remove small amounts of aluminium by conventional dialysis, but in practice the amounts removed compared with the total body burden are likely to be very small. Nevertheless, the clinical improvement which may follow suggests a tiny fraction of the aluminium load may be critically important in determining the immediate toxic manifestations.

Currently, the only method available for removing substantial quantities of aluminium is by chelation with desferrioxamine (DFO). In vitro experiments [*J.P. Day, F.M. Garstang, R.A. Romero*, unpublished observations] have shown that aluminium binds strongly to DFO ($K = 10^{22}$) in a 1:1 molar ratio and its dialysance is consistent with a molecular weight of approximately 600 daltons. This high degree of binding explains why the very high serum aluminium levels achieved following DFO administration appear to cause little toxicity [2]. The amount of aluminium removed during dialysis is related to the prevailing blood level and will be determined by the characteristics of the dialyser. The acute rise in serum aluminium levels following DFO administration indicates mobilisation of aluminium from the tissues and we have demonstrated that aluminium can be removed from both bone trabeculae and bone marrow by repeated DFO administration [3]. The striking clinical improvement and profound histological changes demonstrated have been confirmed by others [4, 5]. Whether these effects are due solely to aluminium removal is uncertain. Other elements also bind strongly to DFO including iron, zinc, copper, chromium and vanadium. However, preliminary studies have failed to show significant removal of any of these elements, apart from iron, from any of our patients.

The side effects of DFO during its use for iron chelation include allergic reactions, abdominal pain, posterior cataracts and retinal changes similar to those seen in retinitis pigmentosa. These, to our knowledge, have not been reported during aluminium chelation, probably due to the lower doses used but this could become relevant in the treatment of children. We have seen exacerbation of bone pain following DFO administration and, more importantly, increased seizure frequency during treatment of severe dialysis encephalopathy.

The place of DFO in the overall strategy of the treatment of aluminium overload has yet to be determined. We believe that DFO is indicated in all cases of clinically apparent encepahlopathy and we have found it particularly helpful during acute encephalopathy following unsuccessful transplantation. Its use in the treatment of severe bone disease appears safe and together with the use of vitamin D, seems to offer the prospect of bone healing and reduction of hypercalcaemia. There may also be a case for its use in patients known to have a significant body burden prior to admission to the transplant waiting list. We speculate that in patients where it is impossible to control hyperphosphataemia without aluminium-containing binders, it may be possible to use DFO intermittently to minimise aluminium accumulation.

References

1   Hodge, K.C.; Day, J.P.; O'Hara, M.; Ackrill, P.; Ralston, A.J.: Critical concentration of aluminium in water used for dialysis. Lancet *ii*: 802–803 (1981).
2   Ackrill, P.; Ralston, A.J.; Day, J.P.; Hodge, K.C.: Successful removal of aluminium from a patient with dialysis encephalopathy. Lancet *i*: 692–693 (1980).
3   Ackrill, P.; Day, J.P.; Garstang, F.M.; Hodge, K.C.; Metcalfe, P.J.; Benzo, Z.; Hill, K.; Ralston, A.J.; Ball, J.; Denton, J.: Treatment of fracturing renal osteodystrophy by desferrioxamine. Proc. Eur. Dial. Transplant. Ass. *19*: 203–207 (1982).
4   Brown, D.J.; Dawborn, J.K.; Ham, K.N.; Xipell, J.M.: Treatment of dialysis osteomalacia with desferrioxamine. Lancet *ii*: 343–345 (1982).
5   Ihle, B.U.; Buchana, M.R.C.; Stevens, B.; Becker, G.J.; Kincaid-Smith, P.: The efficacy of various treatment modalities on aluminium associated bone disease. Proc. Eur. Dial. Transplant, Ass. *19*: 195–201 (1982).

P. Ackrill, MD, Department of Chemistry, Manchester University and Withington Hospital, Manchester M20 8LR (UK)

Contr. Nephrol., vol. 38, pp. 81–91 (Karger, Basel 1984)

Prophylaxis and Methods for Early Recognition of Aluminium Intoxication

C. Fuchs[a], V.W. Armstrong[a], E. Quellhorst[b], F. Scheler[a]

[a]Medical University Clinic of Göttingen, and [b]Nephrologisches Zentrum Niedersachsen, Hann.-Münden, FRG

Introduction

The prophylaxis of aluminium intoxication would be easy if aluminium loading of the organism could be avoided. This is, however, not yet possible. Early recognition of aluminium intoxication is also not feasible because the first clinical signs are manifest only when the aluminium burden has reached an advanced stage. There are no clinical symptoms for the initial phase of an aluminium overload of the organism.

From the practical standpoint, it is therefore important to determine how such an aluminium overload can be avoided and, if it has taken place, which parameters might be valuable to indicate the beginning of an aluminium overload.

Even if aluminium intoxication is reflected by certain neurological symptoms or by special forms of osteomalacia, these disorders are caused by several factors and cannot be controlled and measured as often as a clinical follow-up would demand. In clinical practice the measurement of the plasma aluminium concentration only, would appear to be a useful parameter for long-term observation.

Thus it is the aim of this paper to give some recommendations on the risk of aluminium intoxication due to different dialysis modalities and on the frequency of plasma aluminium control depending on the type of treatment.

Sources of Aluminium Intoxication

The first step in the prophylaxis of aluminium intoxication is to consider possible sources of aluminium overload in renal insufficiency. These would include the aluminium concentration in drinking water, the modality of the water and dialysate preparation, and the phosphate binders or other aluminium-containing drugs that the patient may have to take.

Aluminium in drinking water can affect the aluminium balance of the organism in two ways. One would expect that a high aluminium concentration in drinking water due to local geographical conditions will lead to higher alimentary aluminium ingestion. In addition, further manipulation of the community water supply may be fatal for dialysis patients. *Dunea* et al. [2] described an outbreak of dialysis dementia after the city of Chicago had altered its method of water purification which resulted in higher aluminium levels. 19 patients died. The dialysate aluminium concentrations were around 400 µg/l.

Such events may be fatal if dialysis is performed without reverse osmosis, as is often the case in home hemodialysis. Consequently the responsible centers must regularly check the drinking water and dialysate aluminium concentration in order to decide whether the patients need reverse osmosis water preparation.

For in-center dialysis, a reverse osmosis water preparation should be mandatory. This is particularly important if the community water supply switches from one origin to another. One cannot expect that communities take any responsibility for constant low aluminium contents of the drinking water.

Aluminium Transfer during Dialysis

Graf et al. [8], *Kaehny* et al. [9] and our own hemofiltration data indicate that about 80% of plasma aluminium is protein-bound, whereas 20% is ultrafiltrable or diffusible. *Gitelman* [7] has shown that a high dialysate aluminium content (300 µg/l) maintains high plasma aluminium levels, whereas a low dialysate aluminium concentration (30 µg/l) has a positive influence on plasma levels. Aluminium balance in hemodialysis depends mainly on the gradient of diffusible aluminium; in addition the character of the dialysate membrane, its surface and thickness will also play a role, as well as the duration of treatment. Unfortunately there are no systematic investigations in this field, probably because of the methodological problems involved in carrying out accurate aluminium determinations in dialysate and biological fluids [3].

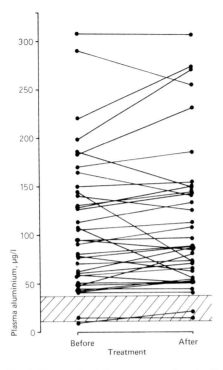

Fig. 1. Plasma aluminium concentrations in 37 hemodialysis patients before and after treatment.

The estimation or interpretation of aluminium transfer during hemodialysis is even more difficult if the influence of the dialysate pH is considered. *Gacek* et al. [4] showed that at a neutral pH aluminium exists as a virtually insoluble hydroxide; small pH shifts in either direction increase aluminium solubility and therefore its diffusibility. This phenomenon should be subjected to a more systematic investigation, especially considering the increased use of bicarbonate dialysis.

At present in the absence of such further investigations, one must recommend dialysate aluminium values not exceeding 10–15 µg/l. Thus hemodialysis patients with plasma aluminium concentrations of 50 µg/l will be protected from a further aluminium load due to dialysis modality. In order to achieve such low dialysate aluminium values, the dialysate concentrate also has to be investigated because the aluminium content of the substances used may vary over a broad range.

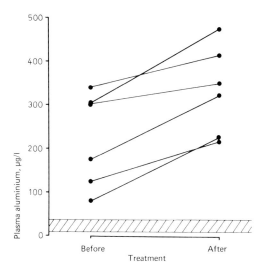

Fig. 2. Plasma aluminium concentrations in 6 Redy® dialysis patients before and after treatment.

On the other hand, we have to realize that even reverse osmosis water preparation leading to an aluminium dialysate concentration below 10 µg/l is no guarantee for low plasma aluminium concentrations.

In Göttingen and in Hann.-Münden plasma aluminium concentrations in 42 center-hemodialysis patients were investigated (fig. 1). Both centers use reverse osmosis for water preparation and the dialysate aluminium concentrations were lower than 8 µg/l. Figure 1 shows some extremely high aluminium concentrations which are not significantly influenced by the low dialysate aluminium. On the basis of these data other possible sources of aluminium uptake must exist.

In addition to single-pass dialysis, recirculation dialysis is also employed in the form of the Redy® cartridge. Figure 2 shows a significant increase in plasma aluminium levels of 6 patients undergoing Redy dialysis.

On testing for aluminium in the dialysate (fig. 3), extremely high dialysate aluminium concentrations of between 227 and 850 µg/l were found before the start of recirculation. On beginning dialysis, the cartridge functioned as an aluminium catcher for a certain period of time. At the end of the 6-hour treatment, however, aluminium was obviously set free again. Unfortunately we did not measure the dialysate pH at that time. *Branger* et al. [1] claim that the aluminium set free would be less if an acetate buffer

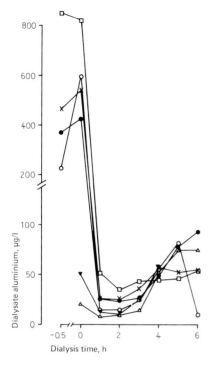

Fig. 3. Dialysate aluminium concentrations before, during, and after Redy® dialysis.

is used instead of bicarbonate, as we used in our investigations. Finally *Odell* et al. [10] have published some data on aluminium kinetics using a new Redy cartridge which seem encouraging.

In hemofiltration, aluminium balance studies are much easier to perform (fig. 4). 20% of the plasma aluminium is ultrafiltrable. Figure 4 documents this linear relation over a broad plasma concentration range. If the disposable materials, that is filter and tubing, are aluminium free the aluminium balance should depend only on the aluminium concentration of the substitution fluid. Several commercially available substitution fluids were investigated. The aluminium concentrations were below 10 µg/l, values which should not harm the patients. A negative aluminium balance with hemofiltration is only possible if there are high plasma values and even in this situation the amount of aluminium removed is minimal. Thus it is not surprising that the plasma aluminium concentrations remain unchanged under hemofiltration treatment (fig. 5). These investigations were performed in 12 patients.

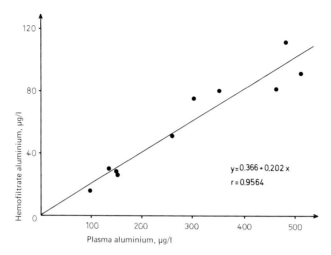

Fig. 4. Correlation of aluminium values in plasma vs. hemofiltrate.

Another 19 patients from the chronic peritoneal dialysis program were investigated. Within this dialysis modality there are two possibilities of dialysate preparation. One is a dialysate preparation by reverse osmosis and mixing with a glucose-electrolyte concentrate; the other is the application of commercially manufactured solutions filled in plastic bags or containers. Both methods of dialysate application were tested. There was no difference between the dialysate aluminium concentrations which showed a mean value of 6.4 μg/l and a maximum of 20 μg/l. Thus one would not expect a serious aluminium load in these patients. The slight increase of the serum levels from 76 to 88 μg/l might be due to hemoconcentration (fig. 6).

Gilli et al. [5, 6] have performed peritoneal dialysate aluminium measurements in the inflow and outflow. In contrast to our findings the dialysate aluminium concentrations were higher, resulting in a positive aluminium balance. In this context the possibility of pH influence should also be considered. It is well known that the peritoneal dialysate solutions are more acidic than hemodialysate solutions.

Finally continuous ambulatory peritoneal dialysis (CAPD) balance studies should be as easy as in hemofiltration, as long as the dialysate used is aluminium free. One should keep in mind the experience of *Winney* et al. [11], who detected CAPD dialysate aluminium concentrations of 1,500

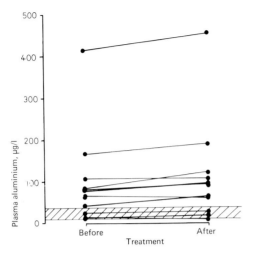

Fig. 5. Plasma aluminium concentrations in 12 hemofiltration patients before and after treatment.

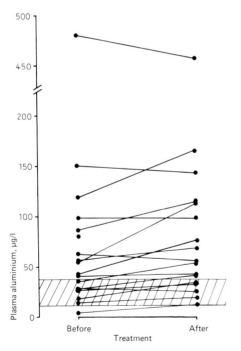

Fig. 6. Serum aluminium concentrations in 19 patients on the intermittent peritoneal dialysis program.

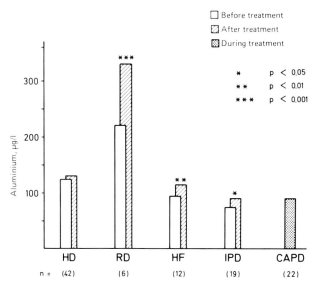

Fig. 7. Plasma or serum aluminium concentrations in 101 chronic renal insufficient patients before, during, and/or after treatment with different modalities. HD = Hemodialysis; RD = Redy dialysis; HF = hemofiltration; IPD = intermittent peritoneal dialysis; CAPD = continuous ambulatory peritoneal dialysis.

µg/l in Edinburgh. The patients had nausea, vomiting, general malaise and colicky abdominal pain. After removing these aluminium-contaminated bags the clinical symptoms subsided.

Figure 7 summarizes the plasma aluminium levels of patients treated by different dialysis modalities. There was a significant increase in Redy® dialysis only due to the dialysis regime. As long as the dialysate aluminium concentrations do not exceed 10–15 µg/l, there is no evidence for a positive aluminium balance due to the different dialysis procedures. The elevated plasma aluminium levels, however, demonstrated here remain unexplained.

Further Sources of Aluminium Overload

In this context one should warn against the use of solutions for parenteral application which are manufactured in the hospitals' own pharmacy without controlling aluminium concentrations (table I).

Table I. Aluminium concentration of solutions manufactured in a hospital's own pharmacy for parenteral application in dialysis treatment in comparison with a commercial solution

Solution	Aluminium concentration µg/l
Hospital	
Glucose, 5%	39
NaCl, 0.9%	52
NaCl, 0.9%	146
Ringer's lactate	760
Commercial	
NaCl, 0.9%	10

Patients at a dialysis center in Lower Saxony had relatively high plasma aluminium concentrations and the source of intoxication was therefore investigated. The dialysate prepared by reverse osmosis and aluminium levels were acceptable (15 µg/l). Thus different solutions were tested which were used for parenteral application in dialysis patients and which were manufactured in the hospital pharmacy (fig. 7). In contrast to a commercial solution, extremely high aluminium concentrations of up to 760 µg/l were detected in the non-commercial solutions.

Commercial plasma albumin solutions have also been found to have aluminium concentrations of up to 900 µg/l.

There is no doubt that a significant source of aluminium load in dialysis patients is the use of aluminium-containing phosphate binders. Dialysis patients consume kilograms of aluminium during the course of renal insufficiency and a certain percentage of this aluminium is bio-available. The intestinal aluminium absorption in renal insufficiency will depend on the acidity of the gastric juice, stomach motility, electrolyte interaction and hormonal influence. Systematic investigations are needed to learn more about this source of aluminium intoxication. At present alternatives to aluminium hydroxide drugs are needed as well as a reduction in their use. Prophylaxis of aluminium toxicity syndrome in the broader sense would then mean that patients should not be subjected to high positive phosphate balances. Physicians should therefore control dietary phosphate intake and they should prefer dialysis procedures with a high phosphate clearance. Probably slightly elevated serum phosphate levels should be accepted if aluminium hydroxide can thus be avoided.

Summarizing Remarks

The prophylaxis of aluminium toxicity syndrome requires the minimization of the aluminium load; that is aluminium-containing drugs should be used as little as possible and dialysis modalities with high phosphate clearance are preferable. The aluminium concentration in dialysate, substitution fluid, electrolyte solution and plasma albumin should not exceed 15 μg/l. Frequent patient control for early recognition of aluminium overload is mandatory. A neurological status should be performed once a year. In hospital dialysis, when using a reverse osmosis water preparation, the patients' plasma aluminium levels should be tested every 3 months and the dialysate aluminium concentration monthly. In home treatment, using reverse osmosis water preparation, patients should be monitored when they come for ambulatory control. At the same time the water and dialysate should be tested. This kind of monitoring should be performed more frequently if fluctuations in the main water supply occur or if no reverse osmosis water preparation is used.

All these recommendations are useless if there is no clinical interpretation of the elevated plasma aluminium concentrations. Plasma levels below 20 μg/l should be considered as being within the normal range. Concentrations from 60 to 100 μg/l should cause no concern since the patient is in no danger of aluminium toxicity. Concentrations over 100 μg/l should cause some concern and would require more careful clinical monitoring. Serum aluminium concentrations of over 200 μg/l should be avoided since clinical symptoms are to be expected.

Finally the better understanding of the aluminium toxicity syndrome in renal insufficiency will depend on sufficient analytical capacity. Thus more laboratories should be equipped to reliably measure aluminium in dialysate and in biological fluids.

References

1　Branger, B.; Ramperez, P.; Marigliano, N.; Mion, H.; Shaldon, S.; Mion, C.: Aluminium transfer in bicarbonate dialysis using a sorbent regenerative system; an in vitro study. Proc. Eur. Dial. Transpl. Ass. *17*: 213−218 (1980).

2　Dunea, G.; Mahurkar, S.D.; Mandani, B.; Smith, E.C.: Role of aluminium in dialysis dementia. Ann. intern. Med. *88*: 502−504 (1978).

3　Fuchs, C.; Brasche, M.; Paschen, K.; Nordbeck, H.; Quellhorst, E.: Aluminiumbestimmung im Serum mit flammenloser Atomabsorption. Clinica chim. Acta *52*: 71−80 (1974).

4   Gacek, E.M.; Babb, A.L.; Urelli, D.A.; Fry, D.L.; Scribner, B.H.: Dialysis dementia: the role of dialysate pH in altering the dializability of aluminium. Trans. Am. Soc. artif. internal Organs 25: 409 (1979).

5   Gilli, P.; de Bastiani, P.; Fagioli, F.; Buoncristiani, U.; Carobi, C.; Stabellini, N.; Squerzanti, R.; Rosati, G.; Farinelli, A.: Postive aluminium balance in patients on regular peritoneal treatment: an effect of low dialysate pH? Proc. Eur. Dial. Transpl. Ass. 17: 219−225 (1980).

6   Gilli, P.; Farinelli, A.; Fagioli, F.; de Bastiani, P.; Buoncristiani, U.: Serum aluminium levels in patients on peritoneal dialysis. Lancet ii: 742−743 (1980).

7   Gitelman, H.: Aluminium measurements in hemodialysis patients and epidemiology. CEC-IUPAC International Workshop on the role of biological monitoring in the prevention of aluminium toxicity in man: aluminium analysis in biological fluids, Luxembourg 1982.

8   Graf, H.; Stummvoll, H.K.; Meister, V.; Kovarik, J.; Wolf, A.; Pinggera, W.F.: Aluminium removal by hemodialysis. Kidney int. 19: 587−592 (1981).

9   Kaehny, W.D.; Alfrey, A.C.; Holman, R.E.; Shorr, W.J.: Aluminium transfer during hemodialysis. Kidney int. 12: 361−365 (1977).

10   Odell, R.A.; Yong, J.; George, C.R.; Farell, P.C.: Aluminium kinetics during sorbent (Redy) dialysis. Contemp. Dial. 3: 57 (1982).

11   Winney, R.J.; Cowie, J.F.; Cumming, A.D.; Rolson, J.S.: Plasma aluminium monitoring in the detection of aluminium toxicity in patients treated by haemodialysis and CAPD. CEC-IUPAC International Workshop on the role of biological monitoring in the prevention of aluminium toxicity in man: aluminium analysis in biological fluids. Luxembourg 1982.

Prof. Dr. med. C. Fuchs, Medical University Clinic of Göttingen,
Robert-Koch-Strasse 40, D-3400 Göttingen (FRG)

Contr. Nephrol., vol. 38, pp. 92–94 (Karger, Basel 1984)

Discussion: Aluminium Metabolism

The questions concerning the paper given by *Cornelis* were mainly related to technical problems: one question referred to the quality control for the dialysate concentrate, which is not generally available, but should be one of the tasks of the Bureau of Reference Materials. *Drüeke* (Paris) raised the issue whether or not special vials or special rubbers should be used for collecting the different samples. *Cornelis* stressed firstly the importance of the time factor as water with an aluminium content of below 100 µg/l should be analyzed within 24 h. Freezing is not as advisable as keeping the sample between 4 and 10 °C. Vials and rubbers of a very high purity are especially desirable for a low aluminium concentration, whereas the risk of contamination in samples with a high aluminium content (above 200 µg/l) is low. With regard to a question from *Pierides* (Rochester) concerning the determination of aluminium in urine, *Cornelis* indicated the difficulties in handling such a heterogenous solution as urine. The discussion of *Savory's* paper was opened by a question concerning the toxicity of the various aluminium fractions, which is not yet clear. In addition, it was stated that the aluminium content of the CSF is very low in spite of high blood levels. *Massry* (Los Angeles) referred in this context to the serum levels of calcium and phosphate, which could be considerably increased without changing their concentration in the CSF. Another issue which was discussed was related to the critical pH which enables the best diffusibility of aluminium. *Savory* stated that there is presently no sufficient data available to forward any recommendations; however, it could be assumed that a pH ranging between 7.2 and 7.6 should be more suitable than a pH below 7.0. *Ritz'* (Heidelberg) question about the influence of various drugs on the partitioning of aluminium could not be answered, as there were no studies available.

Not yet clarified is also the molecular weight of the so-called peak C, which is, according to *Savory*, the dialysable fraction of aluminium. Questions concerning *Knoll*'s paper referred to the gastrointestinal absorption of aluminium. According to *Knoll* there is no sufficient data available with regard to the influence of parathyroid hormone or a normal pH on the uptake of aluminium. However, it seems possible that a normal pH in the gastrointestinal fluid could minimize the absorption of aluminium. Anyhow, intensive examinations in gastrointestinal terms before therapy with aluminium-containing drugs is not justified. The majority of questions raised by *Schneider*'s communication could not be answered satisfactorily by the speaker, because he was obviously not allowed to reveal the secret of the new compound being introduced by him. The discussion of *De Broe*'s paper was opened by a question concerning the localisation of aluminium in the liver, however, only in the lysosomes. *De Broe* underlined the importance of repeated bone biopsies (at least every 2 years), as the aluminium determination in the serum is not very helpful in order to establish the degree of an aluminium intoxication. Furthermore, he mentioned the difficulties of predicting those patients who are at risk in developing such an intoxication as the pathogenesis is multifactorial depending on gastrointestinal uptake, drugs and other not identified conditions. Finally, it was pointed out that it is possibly not sufficient to consider only a lysosomal overload with aluminium in the various organs, but rather to look for special receptors, as even very low concentrations of aluminium can induce severe complications.

Subsequent to *Winney*'s paper, a question was raised concerning the frequency of aluminium determinations in plasma and dialysis fluids. The author recommended controls of plasma aluminium levels in hospital patients every month and in home dialysis patients every 2−3 months. Because of the dangers of acute rises in plasma aluminium levels, especially in younger children on aluminium hydroxide therapy, he claimed that determinations of plasma aluminium levels in those patients were necessary at least at monthly intervals. When asked the reasons for different dialysate aluminium concentrations in different dialysis machines, he speculated that there might be an absorption onto or a release of aluminium from filters inside the dialysis monitors. Supplementing *Cournot-Witmer*'s presentation, *Pierides* confirmed that aluminium has an effect on parathyroid secretion. According to his observation, suppression of parathormone secretion is one of the first signs of aluminium osteopathy characterized by pure osteomalacia.

Following *Pierides'* and *Ackrill's* papers, it was discussed that about a third of the desferrioxamine, injected intravenously, is lost into the gut, thus increasing fecal losses of aluminium and iron. It was mentioned that bone pain disappears after desferrioxamine administration very early after having removed only small amounts of the whole bone aluminium burden. The danger of mental deterioration by increased serum aluminium levels after desferrioxamine application was pointed out.

Prof. *K. Schäfer, Berlin*
Prof. *H.J. Gurland, Munich*

Contr. Nephrol., vol. 38, pp. 95–102 (Karger, Basel 1984)

Zinc Metabolism in Chronic Renal Insufficiency with or without Dialysis Therapy

P.J. Aggett[1]

Royal Aberdeen Children's Hospital and Department of Physiology,
University of Aberdeen, UK

Introduction

Many features of zinc deficiency in laboratory animals and in man resemble some manifestations of chronic renal failure (CRF). In man, zinc-responsive defects include apathy, impaired gustatory and olfactory acuity, anorexia, lethargy, growth retardation, dermatitis, impaired leucocyte chemotaxis, depressed cell-mediated immune function, anaemia, delayed wound healing and diarrhoea. These clinical features and associated biochemical abnormalities have been classically observed in acrodermatitis enteropathica which is probably caused by an inborn error of the intestinal absorption of zinc [1] and in patients on intravenous feeding [2], but the most common cause of inadequate zinc nutrition is protein-energy malnutrition [3]. Experience with these conditions has highlighted the fundamental metabolic importance of zinc and the interdependence of this element with the metabolism of most nutrients. Therefore, although zinc is an essential component for numerous enzyme activities (over 120 in all species), features of zinc deficiency cannot be attributed to loss of specific enzyme functions. Some enzymes are more susceptible to deprivation of zinc than others but, frequently zinc-responsive features, such as loss of affect, anorexia or a check in growth velocity, are apparent before biochemical evidence of zinc deprivation. Zinc has been implemented in the preservation of the integrity of membrane lipids by preventing damage from free

[1] I thank the Rank Prize Fund for financial support.

radicals [4], in essential fatty acid metabolism [5], in microtubular assembly [6] and in the gene expression of *Euglena gracilis* [7]. The features of zinc deficiency are completely non-specific therefore; they can simulate deficiencies of essential fatty acids, essential amino acids and vitamins. It is against this complicated background that one has to consider the metabolism of zinc in CRF and although the more florid manifestations of aerodermatitis enteropathica have not been observed in CRF, there is much evidence that abnormal zinc metabolism is an important factor in this disorder. Some of this evidence will be reviewed.

Zinc Status and Determination of Zinc Content

A constant source of concern in the study of zinc metabolism is that there is no reliable means of determining accurately an individual's nutritional status with respect to the element. The zinc concentrations of hair or of a component of blood, usually plasma, serum or erythrocytes, are used frequently, more because of their convenience than because of their reliability as indicators of zinc status [8]. Futhermore, the import of such values and those derived from other tissue may be limited by several methodological factors. The relative ease and accuracy of quantitative analysis of trace elements in biological tissues and fluids achieved by modern techniques, such as atomic absorption and emission spectroscopy, compared with older colorimetric methods are probably illusory. A valuable review of reported plasma and serum concentrations of zinc as determined by six analytical methods emphasises the variability of results and also the potential errors which accompany sampling procedures [9]. The reported mean plasma zinc concentrations ranged from 0.84 µg/ml (12.9 µmol/l) to 4.28 µg/ml (65.4 µmol/l), most values were between 0.8 and 1.24 µg/ml (12.2–19.0 µmol/l). Serum levels were about 15% higher than plasma values; this has been attributed to release of zinc from haemolysed erythrocytes, its release from platelets during coagulation and to the volume exclusion effect of plasma proteins. More than 0.3% haemolysis of normal red blood cell mass in blood specimens produces discernible increases in plasma and serum zinc concentrations; in uraemia, this margin is even lower because of the higher zinc content of the erythrocytes (see below). The precautions that need to be taken in the sampling, storage and preparation of tissues and biological fluids for analysis have been comprehensively reviewed as have the several analytical methods of determining zinc [10].

Since the hazards of potential contamination and loss of zinc during the preparation of samples are so great and random, the routine use of quality control samples to monitor methodology is desirable. The use of external quality control material provided for interlaboratory comparison and validation would improve confidence in data and would enable the reliable comparison of results from different sources. Unfortunately, few, if any, published reports describing the zinc content of tissue in chronic renal failure provide information about the reproducibility, accuracy and precision of the analyses, and, consequently, the interpretation and comparison of many reports on zinc metabolism in renal disease are limited.

Although low plasma zinc concentrations may indicate suboptimal zinc status they are also caused by factors such as stress, infection, corticosteroids and other endocrine changes [18]. Furthermore, plasma represents less than 0.5% of the total body zinc content. Changes in the zinc content of hair are also induced by factors independent of zinc supply and bear little relation to the zinc content of plasma or soft tissues. In long-term or epidemiological studies, hair may be of some value but, in general, interpretation of hair data is difficult especially since hair zinc content may even be increased in severe zinc deficiency.

The selection of other appropriate tissues as markers of zinc status is under constant review. Skin and bone represent about half of the human zinc content but the turnover of zinc in these tissues, as in hair, is slow. The zinc content of the liver and muscles decrease with zinc deprivation but the decline in the latter is unreliable. Currently, the zinc content of the leucocyte is being explored as an indicator of zinc nutriture, but this may be of limited value in the growing animal, in which deprivation of zinc rapidly impairs growth and much of the smaller amount of new tissue being synthesised maintains a normal zinc content. This further illustrates the point that determination of gross tissue composition may obscure changes in a much smaller but metabolically vital zinc pool. For this reason, alterations of zinc-dependent biochemical activities have been monitored also, but few zinc metallo-enzymes are rapidly responsive to changes in zinc status; those most susceptible to zinc deprivation include deoxynucleotidyl transferase and alkaline phosphatase. The latter would be of limited use in CRF. In general, the most satisfactory means of establishing inadequate zinc nutriture is to monitor appropriate biochemical indices and the clinical status during zinc supplementation. In these circumstances, zinc-responsive features are strongly suggestive of pre-existent absolute or relative depletion of the element.

'Zinc Status' in Chronic Renal Failure

Low plasma or serum zinc levels have been reported in non-dialysed patients with CRF [11−15], but, in dialysed patients, elevated [11, 15], subnormal [12, 14, 15] and almost normal [13] concentrations have been described. Furthermore, some studies have shown appreciable increments of plasma or serum zinc concentrations during a dialysis period [11, 16], in other reports this increase is more modest [13, 15] or absent [14]. In these studies, the erythrocyte zinc content was increased [11, 13−15] in non-dialysed uraemic patients. An early report described no alteration in the zinc content of leucocytes in uraemic patients [17] but other studies [14, 18] have described reduced levels in dialysed and non-dialysed patients; in haemodialysed patients, these reduced levels were restored by zinc supplementation [18]. Since this latter observation was accompanied by an improvement in other zinc-dependent functions, it is an indication of zinc depletion in the study population. Other supplementation studies are described below. The lowered plasma levels could reflect reduced zinc status or a metabolic reaction to the disease state involving altered compartmentalisation of the metal or both [19]. The erythrocyte levels are incompatible with zinc deficiency but it is possible that their accumulation of zinc reflects impaired erythropoiesis due to factors other than zinc deprivation.

The zinc content of tissues derived at autopsy from patients with uraemia confirmed an altered distribution of body zinc in CRF [19]. Thus, in comparison with reference data, a marginal reduction of muscle zinc in uraemia was accompanied by increased zinc content in the heart, spleen and liver and, in dialysed patients, in bone. Unfortunately, data on the zinc in the bones of non-dialysed patients were not available. These subjects had a reduced renal content of zinc which could possibly be attributed to the loss of the cortex which is rich in zinc, and to the increased amount of scar tissue in the organs.

Possible Causes of Altered Zinc Metabolism in Uraemia

The pathogenesis of the changed zinc content of the soft tissues and bone described above is not known. I speculate that part of the pattern could be due to the induction, within the spleen and liver, of metallothionein. The precise function of this cytosolic protein in the metabolism of trace metals is unknown [20]; it binds many metals including copper, zinc and cadmium and its content in tissues is increased in response to some stresses, endotoxaemia, leucocyte endogenous mediators and food restriction; these are essentially the same stimuli which cause depression of the plasma zinc concentration. All of these may be operative in non-dialysed patients with CRF but food or protein restriction may be particularly important; for example, laboratory animals on low protein intakes develop low plasma zinc levels which are unresponsive to zinc supplementation [21]; however, it would be unreliable to interpret these plasma levels as evidence of zinc deficiency because they may represent an altered body distribution of zinc associated in part with increased metallothionein synthesis.

The similarity between protein energy malnutrition and uraemia has been commented on frequently. A restricted protein intake unavoidably reduces the intake of zinc as well as of other essential nutrients [3], because the zinc content of refined carbohydrate and other calorie-rich products is low. Furthermore, low dietary protein may reduce the availability of dietary zinc for absorption. The effects of aluminium hydroxide or of cation exchange resins on the bioavailability of dietary zinc have not been reported but it is noteworthy that therapeutic supplements of inorganic iron such as those used in CRF can impair the absorption of zinc. It has been suggested that depressed 1,25-dihydroxycholecalciferol production also may impair zinc absorption in CRF, but in one study, the effect of this hormone on plasma zinc content was negligible [22], nevertheless, by giving, orally, pharmacological doses of zinc (50 mg) and monitoring the subsequent increments in plasma zinc, *Antoniou* et al. [23] have noted improved intestinal absorption of zinc following therapy with 1,25-hydroxycholecalciferol.

Blood losses during haemodialysis may increase loss of endogenous zinc; and loss of endogenous protein during chronic ambulatory peritoneal dialysis with the net catabolism of tissues in CRF would be expected to release zinc from soft tissue pools. It is conceivable that this zinc may be excreted or sequestered in another pool such as bone. This mechanism could explain the high bone content of zinc noted above and it is an important consideration, therefore, that because bone zinc is poorly mobilised, the metal could become a limiting nutrient even though the crude total body content of zinc may be normal or elevated. Since the demands for zinc are greatest during net anabolism, it is evident that any deficiency of zinc is effectively relative to the general metabolic status of the patients and that zinc-responsive defects may not be apparent until new tissue is being synthesized. This may explain the apparent inconsistency amongst studies of zinc supplementation in CRF which may also illustrate the fact that other essential nutrients are compromised in CRF. Resolution of associated defects may be responsible for increased plasma zinc levels following haemodialysis but, as was mentioned above, this is a variable feature. One potential source of zinc during dialysis is the haemodialysis equipment itself. *Bogden* et al. [24] have noted that zinc uptake from coils ranges from 3.2 to 23.0 mg per dialysis according to the batch of coils. *Mahajan* et al. [14] who used different equipment did not find this phenomenon, and the increasing use of hollow-fibre and parallel-plate dialysers may eliminate this potentially important accessory source of zinc.

Zinc-Responsive Defects in Chronic Renal Failure

Double-blind studies of zinc supplementation in uraemic patients on haemodialysis have shown improved taste acuity and increased dietary intakes of protein and calories following supplementation [25, 26]. Other studies have investigated the effect of zinc supplementation on cell-mediated immunity. One group found anergy to an intradermal challenge with mumps antigen in 1 of 9 haemodialysis patients receiving zinc in the dialysate whereas 11 of 16 non-supplemented patients were anergic; treatment with zinc in 4 of the latter improved the response in 3 [25]. In contrast, another study found that zinc supplementation for 6 weeks had no beneficial effect on the anergic response to skin test antigens, and no significant effect on the in vitro lymphoblast response to phytohaemagglutinin except in 1 patient who was possibly more zinc-depleted than the rest [27].

Mahajan et al. [18] found that when zinc supplements were given to haemodialysis patients, their plasma, leucocyte and hair zinc contents returned to normal, as did their impaired taste function. Supplements were given for 6 months and during this time, elevated plasma ammonia levels fell to the normal range and plasma ribonuclease activity, which is elevated in zinc deficiency, fell but did not reach normal levels of activity. Of these indices the leucocyte zinc content was the first to show any response to zinc. These observations were made on patients with dietary protein intakes of 60 g or more a day which should have provided an adequate amount of dietary zinc, and they emphasize the need to investigate further the cause of apparent zinc depletion in chronic renal failure, and to stimulate the study of other aspects of this disorder which may respond to zinc. Impaired sexual function and the possible role of zinc deficiency will be discussed later. Other aspects such as platelet aggregation, the metabolism of lipids, water and prostaglandins, and membrane function as well as endocrine and other nutritional abnormalities are of interest. However, it is important in all these studies to consider the possibility that one is observing a pharmacological rather than a physiological effect, whereby effects attributed to zinc may be due to correction of other defects induced by improved appetite and general nutrition.

References

1 Aggett, P.J.: Acrodermatitis enteropathica. J. inherit metab. Dis. 6: 39–43, suppl. 1 (1983).

2 Kay, R.G.; Tasman-Jones, C.; Pybus, J.; Whiting, R.; Black, H.: A syndrome of acute zinc deficiency during total parenteral alimentation in man. Ann. Surg. 183: 331–340 (1976).

3 Golden, M.H.N.; Golden, B.E.: Trace elements. Potential importance in human nutrition with particular reference to zinc and vanadium. Br. med. Bull. 37: 31–36 (1981).

4 Editorial: A radical approach to zinc. Lancet i: 191 (1978).

5 Bettger, W.J.; O'Dell, B.L.: Minireview. A critical physiological role of zinc in the structure and function of biomembranes. Life Sci. 28: 1425–1438 (1981).

6 Hesketh, J.E.: Impaired microtubule assembly in brain from zinc deficient pigs and rats. Int. J. Biochem. 13: 921–926 (1981).

7 Vallee, B.L.; Falchuk, K.H.: Zinc and gene expression. Phil. Trans. R. Soc. 294: 185–197 (1981).

8 Solomons, N.W.: On the assessment of zinc and copper nutriture in man. Am. J. clin. Nutr. 32: 856–871 (1979).

9 Versieck, J.; Cornelis, R.: Normal levels of trace elements in human blood or serum. Analytica chim. Acta 116: 217–254 (1980).

10 Elemental analysis of biological materials. Techn. Rep. Ser., No. 197 (International Atomic Energy Agency, Vienna 1980).

11 Rose, G.A.; Willden, E.G.: Whole blood, red cell and plasma total and ultrafiltrable zinc levels in normal subjects and patients with chronic renal failure with and without haemodialysis. Br. J. Urol. 44: 281–286 (1972).

12 Condon, C.J.; Freeman, R.M.: Zinc metabolism in renal failure. Ann. intern. Med. 73: 531–536 (1970).

13 Mansouri, K.; Halsted, J.A.; Gombos, E.A.: Zinc, copper, magnesium and calcium in dialysed and non-dialysed uremic patients. Archs intern. Med. 125: 88–93 (1970).

14 Mahajan, S.K.; Prasad, A.S.; Rabbani, P.; Briggs, W.A.; McDonald, F.D.: Zinc metabolism in uraemia. J. Lab. clin. Med. 94: 693–698 (1979).

15 Mahler, D.J.; Walsh, J.R.; Haynie, G.D.: Magnesium, zinc and copper in dialysis patients. Am. J. clin. Path. 56: 17–23 (1971).

16 Bogden, J.D.; Oleske, J.M.; Weiner, B.; Smith, L.G., Jr.; Smith, L.G.; Najem, G.R.: Elevated plasma zinc concentrations in renal dialysis patients. Am. J. clin. Nutr. 33: 1088–1095 (1980).

17 Michael, J.; Hilton, P.J.; Jones, N.F.: Zinc and the sodium pump in uremia. Am. J. clin. Nutr. *31*: 1945–1947 (1978).

18 Mahajan, S.K.; Prasad, A.S.; Rabbani, P.; Briggs, W.A.; McDonald, F.D.: Zinc deficiency: a reversible complication of uremia. Am. J. clin. Nutr. *36*: 1177–1183 (1982).

19 Smythe, W.R.; Alfrey, A.C.; Craswell, P.W.; Crouch, C.A.; Ibels, L.S.; Kubo, H.; Nunnelley, L.L.; Rudolph, H.: Trace element abnormalities in chronic uremia. Ann. intern. Med. *96*: 302-310 (1982).

20 Webb, M.; Cain, K.: Functions of metallothionein. Biochem. Pharmac. *31*: 137–142 (1982).

21 Filteau, S.M.; Woodward, B.: The effect of severe protein deficiency on serum zinc concentration of mice fed a requirement level or a very high level of dietary zinc. J. Nutr. *112*: 1974–1977 (1982).

22 Kiilerich, S.; Christiansen, C.; Christiansen, M.S.; Naestoft, J.: Zinc metabolism in patients with chronic renal failure during treatment with 1,25-dihydroxycholecalciferol: a controlled therapeutic trial. Clin. Nephrol. *15*: 23–27 (1981).

23 Antoniou, L.D.; Shalhoub, R.J.; Elliot, S.: Zinc tolerance tests in chronic uremia. Clin. Nephrol. *16*: 181–187 (1981).

24 Bodgen, J.D.; Zadzielski, E.; Weiner, B.; Oleske, J.M.; Aviv, A.: Release of some trace methods from disponsible coils during haemodialysis. Am. J. clin. Nutr. *36*: 403–409 (1982).

25 Atkin-Thor, E.; Goddard, B.W.; O'Nion, J.; Stephen, R.L.; Kolff, W.J.: Hypogeusia and zinc depletion in chronic dialysis patients. Am. J. clin. Nutr. *31*: 1948–1951 (1978).

26 Mahajan, S.K.; Prasad, A.S.; Lambujon, J.; Abbasi, A.A.; Briggs, W.A.; McDonald, F.D.: Improvement of uremic hypogeusia by zinc: a double-blind study. Am. J. clin. Nutr. *33*: 1517–1521 (1980).

27 Antoniou, L.D.; Shalhoub, R.J.; Schecter, G.P.: The effect of zinc on cellular immunity in chronic uremia. Am. J. clin. Nutr. *34*: 1912–1917 (1981).

28 Allen, J.I.; Korchik, W.; Kay, N.E.; McClain, C.J.: Zinc and T-lymphocyte function in haemodialysis patients. Am. J. clin. Nutr. *36*: 410–415 (1982).

Dr. P.J. Aggett, Department of Physiology, Marischal College,
University of Aberdeen, Aberdeen AB9 1AS (UK)

Contr. Nephrol., vol. 38, pp. 103–111 (Karger, Basel 1984)

Sexual Dysfunction in Uremic Male: Improvement Following Oral Zinc Supplementation

Sudesh K. Mahajan, Ananda S. Prasad, Franklin D. McDonald

Department of Medicine, Veterans Administration Medical Center, Allen Park, Mich. USA; Wayne State University, School of Medicine, Detroit, Mich., USA

Abnormalities of sexual function [1–7] and zinc metabolism [8–10] have been reported in patients with chronic renal failure and are not improved by maintenance hemodialysis therapy. The factors underlying sexual dysfunction in uremia are not clear. The presence of psychological instability [1–5], gonadal dysfunction [11–13], hyperparathyroidism [14, 15] and hyperprolactinemia [16] have been implicated. Recent studies have suggested that sexual dysfunction in uremic males may be related to abnormal zinc metabolism in these patients [17–20]. Since the purpose of this report is to assess influences of zinc on sexual dysfunction in chronic renal failure, we will confine our remarks to the available evidence in regard to zinc deficiency as a possible cause of sexual dysfunction in uremia.

In order to establish a casual relationship between zinc deficiency and sexual dysfunction, one must address the following issues: (1) Zinc deficiency is present in chronic renal failure. (2) Sexual dysfunction has an organic basis. (3) Gonadal dysfunction is the cause of sexual dysfunction. (4) Reversal of zinc deficiency and gonadal dysfunction by zinc supplementation. (5) Normalization of gonadal function improves sexual dysfunction.

Zinc Deficiency in Uremia

The criteria for the diagnosis of zinc deficiency in humans are not well established. Among the available laboratory parameters, determination of plasma or serum zinc has been the most widely used to assess zinc status. These values, although constant in the state of good health, are known to fluctuate markedly in situations of stress, including chronic renal failure [21]. Subnormal plasma zinc levels have been reported in patients with chronic renal failure [8–10]. However, their significance as an index of zinc deficiency in uremia is doubtful since they have also been reported to be normal [22] and high [23] in uremia. In order to critically evaluate the zinc status in patients with chronic renal failure, we determined zinc concentrations in plasma, hair and leukocytes as well as the plasma activity of the zinc-dependent enzyme ribonuclease and plasma ammonia, in patients undergoing hemodialysis and peritoneal dialysis and in nondialyzed uremic patients. All patients had subnormal concentrations of zinc in plasma, hair and leukocytes as well as increased plasma ribonuclease and plasma ammonia [10]. Similar biochemical changes have been reported in experimentally induced zinc deficiency in both animals and man [24]. This constellation of biochemical parameters of abnormal zinc metabolism are suggestive, but not diagnostic, of zinc deficiency in uremia.

Since a favorable response to zinc supplementation is considered to be a reliable index of zinc deficiency in humans, we initiated a double-blind study using oral zinc supplementation with zinc acetate (50 mg of elemental zinc per day) or placebo. 24 stable patients with end stage renal disease undergoing maintenance hemodialysis for more than 6 months completed the study. The study was terminated after 6 months. Zinc concentration in plasma, hair and leucocytes as well as plasma ammonia and plasma ribonuclease were measured before, and every 6 weeks after, starting the treatment. Only patients receiving zinc demonstrated significant increases in plasma zinc, hair zinc and leukocyte zinc as well as decreases in plasma ribonuclease and plasma ammonia [25]. Inasmuch as all other variables, including dietary protein intake, medications and dialysis treatment remained the same, it is reasonable to assume that biochemical improvements noted were related to reversal of zinc deficiency in these patients.

Sexual Dysfunction in Uremia

Sexual function abnormalities including impotence, decreased libido and decreased frequency of intercourse are not uncommon among patients with chronic renal failure. Sexual dysfunction does not improve or may first manifest itself after initiation of maintenance dialysis therapy [1]. The results from questionnaires and structured interviews have shown that total or partial impotence is present in more than 50% of patients with chronic renal failure [1−7]. However, the questionnaires provide only subjective information and lack objective data regarding the incidence, mechanisms and causative factors underlying genesis of sexual dysfunction in uremia. Psychological instability imposed by the chronic illness and the dependency on dialysis were implicated as a cause for uremic impotence in earlier studies [1−5]. The measurement of nocturnal penile tumescence is considered useful for the differentiation between a psychogenic and an organic basis of impotence [26]. The finding of abnormal nocturnal penile tumescence in 8 of 11 symptomatic patients by *Parker* et al. [6] and in 22 of 48 patients by *Procci* et al. [7] suggests an organic basis for sexual dysfunction in most patients with chronic renal failure. The presence of autonomic insufficiency, peripheral neuropathy, vascular insufficiency, and the use of certain antihypertensive drugs may contribute to the severity of uremic impotence.

Gonadal Dysfunction in Uremia

Gonadal dysfunction has been a consistent finding in uremic males [11−18]. The finding of low serum testosterone levels and oligospermia [12, 18] suggest that patients with renal failure are infertile. Impotence and decreased libido may be due to testosterone deficiency in uremia. Impotence in some uremic patients with testosterone in the normal range may be related to decreased conversion of testosterone to an active metabolite such as dihydrotestosterone [17]. Testosterone deficiency in uremia may be due to either hypothalamic-pituitary-testicular dysfunction or direct uremic toxicity on reproductive tissue. Evidence in support of the latter includes impaired spermatogenesis and histologic abnormalities of testicular interstitial cells [12, 13]. The binding capacity and metabolic clearance rate of testosterone are normal in uremia [11]. The hypothalamic-pituitary-testicular axis appears to be normal in uremic males as shown by elevated levels of serum luteinizing hormone (LH) in the presence of low serum testosterone levels and by the normal gonadotrophin response to the administration of clomiphene [12] and trophic hormone [13, 18]. Oligospermia and low serum testosterone levels in the presence of elevated serum follicle-stimulating hormone (FSH) and LH levels in uremic patients suggest primary gonadal failure.

Table I. Results of zinc supplementation studies on gonadal and sexual function in hemodialysis patients

	Antoniou et al. [17] 1977	Zetin [29] 1980	Brook et al. [30] 1980	Mahajan et al. [20] 1982
Number of patients	4	10	7	10
Zinc supplementation				
Route	dialytic	dialytic	dialytic	oral
Dosage	400 µg/l	400 µg/l	400 µg/l	50 mg/day
Duration, months	4	1	1.5	6
Plasma zinc	↑	→	↑	↑
Gonadal functions				
Testosterone	↑	ND	→	↑
LH	↓	ND	→	↓
FSH	↓	ND	→	↓
Sperm counts	ND	ND	ND	↑
Sexual function				
Subjective	↑	→	→	↑
Objective (NPT)	ND	ND	→	ND

↑ = Increased; → = no change; ↓ = decreased from before therapy; ND = not done; NPT = nocturnal penile tumescence.

Elevated blood levels of prolactin and parathyroid hormone (PTH) have been implicated in the pathogenesis of gonadal dysfunction in uremic males [14–16]. It has been suggested that high prolactin levels inhibit the action of gonadotrophic hormones at the gonadal level. Reduction in prolactin levels by bromocriptine has been associated with improvement in sexual dysfunction [27]. The finding of significant correlation between the degree of impotence and the magnitude of secondary hyperparathyroidism by *Loew* et al. [14] and improvement of gonadal function and sexual dysfunction in 7 uremic patients following treatment with $1.25(OH)_2D_3$ by *Massry* et al. [15] suggest that excess blood levels of PTH may play a significant role in the genesis of uremic impotence.

Table II. Plasma zinc levels and gonadal functions in hemodialysis patients before and after oral zinc and placebo therapy

	Controls (n = 20)	Zinc acetate (50 mg/day) (n = 20)		Placebo (n = 20)	
		before	after	before	after
Plasma zinc, μg/dl	106 ± 10	75 ± 2	100 ± 2*	74 ± 2	75 ± 3
Serum testosterone, ng/ml	6.0 ± 1.0	3.0 ± 0.3	5.0 ± 0.5*	3.0 ± 0.3	3.0 ± 0.3
Serum LH, mIU/ml	14 ± 2	92 ± 10	49 ± 26*	40 ± 7	38 ± 8
Serum FSH, mIU/ml	12 ± 3	45 ± 9	25 ± 7*	33 ± 3	35 ± 5
Sperm counts, millions/ml	230 ± 80	30 ± 3	63 ± 5*	32 ± 3	28 ± 3

*$p < 0.005$ from before therapy.

Reversal of Gonadal Dysfunction by Zinc

Zinc is an essential trace element for animals and man. Growth retardation, testicular atrophy, abnormalities of gustation and olfaction, and impaired wound healing have been associated with zinc deficiency in humans and animals [28]. Similar clinical manifestations are also present in uremic patients and are not improved by dialysis [10]. *Antoniou* et al. [17] were the first to show the beneficial effect of zinc supplementation on gonadal dysfunction. They found that dialytic administration of zinc (zinc chloride 400 μg/l) but not zinc sulfate orally (150 mg of elemental zinc per day) for 4 months was able to reverse gonadal dysfunction in their patients (table I). Similarly designed studies by *Zetin and Stone* [29] and *Brooks* et al. [30] failed to demonstrate the beneficial effect of zinc on gonadal function (table I). The short duration of therapy (4–6 weeks) may explain the lack of improvement in both studies, although persistence of hypozincemia may explain the therapeutic failure seen by *Zetin and Stone* [29].

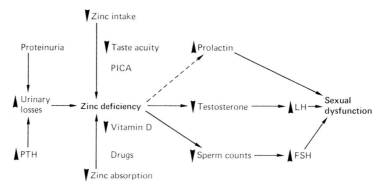

Fig. 1. Factors underlying zinc deficiency, gonadal function and sexual dysfunction in uremia.

To evaluate more critically the possibility that zinc deficiency is a reversible cause of gonadal dysfunction in uremia, we initiated a double-blind study using oral zinc (zinc acetate 50 mg/day) and a placebo. 20 stable hemodialysis patients completed the study. Zinc supplementation but not the placebo brought about normal serum testosterone and sperm counts in all patients after 6 months (table II). Serum LH and FSH levels decreased but remained above the normal range (table II). These results suggest that hormonal evidence of primary gonadal failure persists despite normalization of serum testosterone and sperm counts by zinc therapy. The reason for this disparity in the normal relation between circulating LH and testosterone, and serum FSH levels and sperm counts in our patients is not clear. Zinc acetate in contrast to zinc sulfate was well tolerated on an empty stomach in our patients. In fact, it was not associated with any ill effects in our patients. We suspect that both better compliance and better absorption resulted. Our patients taking zinc acetate had normal plasma zinc levels after 6 months, suggesting that zinc absorption is normal and 50 mg/day is an optimal dosage in hemodialysis patients.

Gonadal Dysfunction and Sexual Dysfunction

Although most studies failed to demonstrate a significant relationship between levels of gonadal hormones and sexual dysfunction, impotence in uremia appears to be due to gonadal dysfunction because normalization of gonadal function following zinc [17, 20], bromocriptine [27], and vitamin D [15] therapy resulted in subjective improvement in sexual potency. Objective assessment of sexual function, such as determining nocturnal penile tumescence before and after therapy, should be done to establish the relationship between gonadal dysfunction and uremic impotence.

It is obvious from the available data that pathogenesis of sexual dysfunction in uremia is not clear. A large-scale comprehensive analysis of various organic and psychological factors and an objective assessment of impotence in dialysis patients is needed to ascertain the true incidence and pathogenesis of, and possible therapeutic approaches to, uremic impotence. It is our opinion that zinc deficiency plays a significant role in the genesis of sexual dysfunction in uremia. The role of zinc on gonadal function is not known. Zinc is essential for nucleic acid synthesis and activities of many enzymes [28]. Zinc concentrations normally high in kidneys, prostate and testes are reduced in uremia [8]. Zinc deficiency may cause abnormalities in nucleic acid and protein synthesis by these organs. The predominant role of zinc in gonadal function is probably an effect in cellular proliferation.

The cause of zinc deficiency in uremia is not known. Zinc deficiency in uremia may be due to protein calorie malnutrition, dietary habits, decreased bio-availability of zinc in the diet, decreased intestinal absorption of dietary zinc, drug interactions with zinc and increased urinary excretion of zinc (fig. 1). Until the underlying factors of zinc deficiency are ascertained, appropriate caution should be exercised in the use of zinc therapy for sexual dysfunction in uremia. Zinc supplementation is indicated only in those patients who have been proved zinc deficient and in whom other causes of sexual dysfunction have been excluded. We feel that oral zinc supplementation is as effective as dialytic administration of zinc in correcting sexual dysfunction, provided the therapy is continued for at least 6 months.

References

1   Levy, N.B.: Sexual adjustment of maintenance hemodialysis and renal transplantation. National survey by questionnaire: preliminary report. Trans. Am. Soc. artif. internal Organs *19*: 138–143 (1973).

2   Thurm, J.: Sexual potency of patients on chronic hemodialysis. Urology *5*: 60–62 (1975).

3   Levy, N.B.: The quality of life on maintenance hemodialysis. Lancet *i*: 1328–1330 (1975).

4   Sherman, F.P.: Impotence in patients with chronic renal failure on dialysis. Its frequency and etiology. Fert. Steril. 26: 221–223 (1975).

5   Bommer, J.; Tschoepe, W.; Ritz, E.; Andrassy, K.: Sexual behavior of hemodialysis patients. Clin. Nephrol. 6: 315–318 (1976).

6   Parker, R.A.; Bennett, R.M.; Harris, R.L.; Barry, J.; Porter, G.A.: Nocturnal penile tumescence. An objective method for the evaluation of impotence in chronic renal failure. Proc. clin. Dial. Transplant Forum 7: 34–38 (1977).

7   Procci, W.R.; Goldstein, D.A.; Adelstein, J.; Massry, S.G.: Sexual dysfunction in male patients with uremia. A reappraisal. Kidney int. 19: 317–323 (1981).

8   Condon, C.J.; Freeman, R.M.: Zinc metabolism in renal failure. Ann. intern. Med. 73: 531–536 (1970).

9   Lindeman, R.D.; Baxter, D.J.; Yunice, A.A.; Kraikitpanitch, S.: Serum concentrations and urinary excretions of zinc in cirrhosis, nephrotic syndrome and renal insufficiency. Am. J. med. Sci. 275: 17–31 (1979).

10   Mahajan, S.K.; Prasad, A.S.; Rabbani, P.; Briggs, W.A.; McDonald, F.D.: Zinc metabolism in uremia. J. Lab. clin. Med. 94: 693–698 (1979).

11   Stewart-Bently, M.; Gans, D.; Horton, R.: Regulation of gonadal function in uremia. Metabolism 23: 1065–1072 (1974).

12   Lim, V.S.; Fang, V.S.: Gonadal dysfunction in uremic men: A study of the hypothalamopituitary-testicular axis before and after renal transplantation. Am. J. Med. 58: 655–662 (1975).

13   Holdsworth, S.; Atkins, M.B.; DeKrester, D.M.: The pituitary-testicular axis in men with chronic renal failure. New Engl. J. Med. 296: 1245–1249 (1977).

14   Loew, H.; Schultz, H.; Busch, G.: Klinische Aspekte der Impotenz männlicher Dauerdialyzepatienten. Medsche Welt 26: 1651–1652 (1975).

15   Massry, S.G.; Goldstein, D.A.; Procci, W.R.; Kletzky, O.A.: Impotence in patients with uremia. A possible role for parathyroid hormone (Editorial). Nephron 19: 305–310 (1977).

16   Gura, V.; Weizman, A.; Maoz, B.; Zevin, D.; Ben-David, M.: Hyperprolactinemia. A possible cause of sexual impotence in male patients undergoing chronic hemodialysis. Nephron 26: 53–54 (1980).

17   Antoniou, L.D.; Sudhaker, T.; Shalhoub, R.J.; Smith, J.C.: Reversal of uremic impotence by zinc. Lancet ii: 895–898 (1977).

18   Mahajan, S.K.; Abbasi, A.A.; Prasad, A.S.; Briggs, W.A.; McDonald, F.D.: Relationship between uremic hypogonadism and zinc. Proc. clin. Dial. Transplant Forum 9: 165–170 (1979).

19   Mahajan, S.K.; Prasad, A.S.; Briggs, W.A.; McDonald, F.D.: Effect of zinc therapy on sexual dysfunction in hemodialysis patients. Trans. Am. Soc. Artif. Intern. Organs 26: 139–141 (1980).

20   Mahajan, S.K.; Abbasi, A.A.; Prasad, A.S.; Rabbani, P.; Briggs, W.A.; McDonald, F.D.: Effect of oral zinc therapy on gonadal function in hemodialysis patients. A double blind study. Ann. intern. Med. 97: 357–361 (1982).

21   Beisel, W.R.; Pekarek, R.S.: Acute stress and trace element metabolism; in Pfeifer, Neurobiology of the trace metals zinc and copper, pp. 53–82 (Academic Press, New York 1972).

22   Mansouri, K.; Halsted, J.; Gombos, E.A.: Zinc, copper, magnesium and calcium in dialyzed and non-dialyzed uremic patients. Archs. intern. Med. 125: 88–93 (1970).

23   Rose, G.A.; Wilden, E.G.: Whole blood, red cell and plasma total and ultrafilterable
      zinc levels in normal subjects and in patients with chronic renal failure with and without
      hemodialysis. Br. J. Urol. *44*: 281–288 (1972).
24   Prasad, A.S.; Rabbani, P.; Abbasi, A.A.; Bowersox, E.; FoxSpivey, M.R.: Experi-
      mental zinc deficiency in humans. Ann. intern. Med. *89*: 483–490 (1978).
25   Mahajan, S.K.; Prasad, A.S.; Rabbani, P.; Briggs, W.A.; McDonald, F.D.: Zinc defi-
      ciency. A reversible complication of uremia. Am. J. clin. Nutr. *36*: 1177–1183 (1982).
26   Fisher, C.; Schiavi, R.C.; Edwards, A.; Davis, D.M.; Reitman, M.; Fine, Y.: Evalua-
      tion of nocturnal penile tumescence in the differential diagnosis of sexual impotence. A
      quantitative study. Archs. gen. Psychiat. *36*: 431–437 (1979).
27   Bommer, J.; Del-Pozo, E.; Ritz, E.; Bommer, G.: Improved sexual function in male
      hemodialysis patients on bromocriptine. Lancet *ii*: 496–497 (1979).
28   Prasad, A.S.: Zinc in human nutrition. Crit. Rev. clin. Lab. Sci. *8*: 1–80 (1977).
29   Zetin, M.; Stone, R.A.: Effects of zinc in chronic hemodialysis. Clin. Nephrol. *13*:
      20–25 (1980).
30   Brook, A.C.; Johnston, D.G.; Ward, M.K.; Watson, M.J.; Cook, D.B.; Kerr, D.N.S.:
      Absence of a therapeutic effect of zinc in the sexual dysfunction of hemodialysis pa-
      tients. Lancet *ii*: 618–619 (1980).

S.K. Mahajan, MD, Medical Service, V.A. Medical Center,
Allen Park, MI 48101 (USA)

Contr. Nephrol., vol. 38, pp. 112–115 (Karger, Basel 1984)

Zinc Metabolism Does Not Influence Sexual Function in Chronic Renal Insufficiency

R.S.C. Rodger, A.C. Brook, N. Muirhead, D.N.S. Kerr

Department of Medicine, Royal Victoria Infirmary, Newcastle upon Tyne, England

In 1921 *Bertrand and Vladesco* [1] were first to describe high concentrations of zinc in male reproductive organs and suggested that zinc might be important in testicular function. This finding was substantiated 30 years later by *Mawson and Fischer* [2] and led to the experiment by *Millar* et al. [3] in 1958 which demonstrated that male rats fed a zinc-deficient diet developed hypogonadism and testicular atrophy. Finally, in 1963, *Prasad* et al. [4] reported a chronic zinc deficiency syndrome, characterized by poor growth and delayed sexual maturity in adolescent boys which was reversed with zinc replacement. Thus, the association between zinc deficiency and sexual dysfunction was established.

Men with chronic renal failure experience loss of libido, erectile impotence and are usually infertile. This persists and may worsen following the onset of regular dialysis therapy. We have recently interviewed our male dialysis patients using a standard questionnaire including specific questions about sexual activity and frequency of penile erections prior to the onset of renal failure, during chronic renal failure, and once established on regular dialysis. Erectile impotence was present in approximately 80% of patients (table I). This is in keeping with previous reports [5, 6] and suggests that improvements in dialysis therapy have not influenced the frequency of sexual dysfunction in end-stage renal disease.

Although hypozincaemia has consistently been reported in patients with chronic renal failure [7, 8], there is considerable overlap with normal levels. We have measured serum zinc in 58 male dialysis patients (table II) and found it to be low in almost 60% of the cases. Plasma testosterone levels were low in 17% of the patients, but there was no correlation between serum zinc and plasma testosterone levels in our study. Even where zinc

Table I. Erectile impotence in 27 Newcastle dialysis patients 1983

	Partial	Complete	Total
HD, %	18	64	82
CAPD, %	38	38	76

HD = Hemodialysis; CAPD = Continuous ambulatory peritoneal dialysis.

Table II. Newcastle and Sunderland male dialysis patients (HD and CAPD) 1982 (mean ± SE)

	n	Serum zinc (11−25 μmol/l)	Plasma testosterone (8.5−27.5 nmol/l)
HD	38	11.4 ± 2.9	12.6 ± 6.7
CAPD	20	11.2 ± 2.7	14.9 ± 6.7

HD = Hemodialysis; CAPD = Continuous ambulatory peritoneal dialysis.

therapy has been shown to reverse uraemic impotence, there is no correlation between zinc levels and sexual function [9]. Furthermore, the study by *Condon and Freeman* [7] of post mortem tissues in 9 patients with renal failure showed no significant difference in zinc content in heart, liver, or testes from controls. Thus, the interpretation of hypozincaemia in chronic renal failure as a measure of total body zinc status is unreliable, and the response to zinc supplementation remains the standard method to assess zinc deficiency. More recently, *Ribeiro* et al. [10] have shown that uraemic rats had lower plasma testosterone but higher testicular zinc levels than sham-operated controls. He concluded that zinc deficiency is not involved in the pathogenesis of sexual dysfunction in uraemic rats.

The report by *Antoniou* et al. [11] of the reversal of uraemic impotence by zinc prompted our own group to perform a double-blind study of zinc therapy versus placebo on sexual function and endocrine status in renal failure. *Brook* et al. [12] studied 14 male haemodialysis patients, mean age 38 years, who were divided randomly into two groups. Zinc chloride or placebo was added to the dialysate bath for a 6-week period. Sexual func-

tion was assessed by standard questionnaire and nocturnal penile tumescence monitoring (NPTM) for 2–3 nights in the patient's home. Serum
zinc, gonadotrophin, and plasma testosterone values were measured before and after the period of treatment.

After 6 weeks, serum zinc levels were increased significantly in the
zinc-supplemented group, but there was no change in testosterone or
gonadotrophin levels. In neither group was sexual function significantly altered as judged by questionnaire response or NPTM. These patients had
markedly reduced erectile activity during sleep compared with normal controls.

In California, *Zetin and Stone* [13] studied 10 male haemodialysis patients in a double-blind crossover experiment comparing dialytic zinc with
placebo over two 4-week periods. The patients completed questionnaires
assessing depression and sexual activity during the study. There was no correlation between depression rating and sexual dysfunction, and sexual
function did not improve following zinc therapy.

One explanation for the negative results in these studies is that the duration of zinc therapy was too short. However, the original report by *Antoniou* et al. [11] stated that striking benefit was seen after only 2 weeks of
treatment in most patients. *Zetin and Stone* [13] have been further criticised
because their study failed to increase serum zinc levels significantly. This
may be partly explained, by the fact that their data on serum zinc levels
were incomplete. Certainly they used the same dialysate zinc concentration
as *Antoniou* et al. [11] and *Brook* et al. [12].

Mahajan et al. [8, 14] have reported two major studies demonstrating
improvement of sexual function endocrine status and sperm counts after
oral zinc supplementation. The improvement in sexual function was based
on patient questionnaire response which can be unreliable when compared
with NPTM [12] or questionnaire response from the patient's spouse [un-
published observation]. Although plasma testosterone levels increased significantly after zinc therapy, there was no correlation between testosterone
levels and sexual function. This suggests that the free testosterone may
have been unchanged and the apparent increase secondary to a rise in sex
hormone binding globulin which was not measured. Even after therapy
sperm counts remained very low and approximately a quarter of normal
levels.

In order to clarify the role of zinc supplementation in the management
of sexual dysfunction in males with end-stage renal failure, further studies
are needed. Sexual dysfunction in renal failure is multifactorial, and, there-

fore, patients with hyperprolactinaemia, testicular atrophy, vascular and psychogenic impotence, or taking drugs known to cause impotence should be excluded from these trials. NPTM is of value in such research to distinguish organic from psychogenic impotence [15] and to provide a repeatable objective measure of sexual function.

Acknowledgements

We wish to acknowledge the Department of Clinical Chemistry who measured zinc and testosterone levels in our patients and Dr. *M. McHugh* and Dr. *A. Martin* who allowed their patients to be included in our survey. We thank *Deirdre Cook* for secretarial help.

References

1   Bertrand, G.; Vladesco, R.: C. r. *173*: 176 (1921).
2   Mawson, C.A.; Fischer, M.I.: Nature *167*: 859 (1951).
3   Millar, M.J.; Fischer, M.I.; Elcoate, P.V.; Mawson, C.A.: Can. J. Biochem. Physiol. *36*: 557 (1958).
4   Prasad, A.S.; Schulert, A.R.; Miale, A., et al.: J. Lab. clin. Med. *61*: 537 (1963).
5   Abram, H.S.; Hester, L.R.; Sheridan, W.F.; Epstein, G.M.: J. nerv. ment. Dis. *160*: 220 (1975).
6   Procci, W.R.; Goldstein, D.A.; Adelstein, J.; Massry, S.G.: Kidney int. *19*: 317 (1981).
7   Condon, C.J.; Freeman, R.M.: Ann. intern. Med. *73*: 531 (1970).
8   Mahajan, S.K.; Prasad, A.S.; Rabbani, P., et al.: J. Lab. clin. Med. *94*: 693 (1979).
9   Mahajan, S.K.; Abbasi, A.A.; Prasad, A.S., et al.: Ann. intern. Med. *97*: 357 (1982).
10 Ribeiro, R.C.J.; Neves, F.A.R.; Albuquerque, R.H., et al.: Nephron *30*: 361 (1982).
11 Antoniou, L.D.; Shalhoub, R.J.; Sudhaker, T.; Smith, J.C.: Lancet *ii*: 895 (1977).
12 Brook, A.C.; Johnson, D.G.; Ward, M.K., et al.: Lancet *ii*: 618 (1980).
13 Zetin, M.; Stone, R.A.: Clin. Nephrol. *13*: 20 (1980).
14 Mahajan, S.K.; Prasad, A.S.; Briggs, W.A.; McDonald, F.D.: Trans. Am. Soc. artif. internal Organs *26*: 139 (1980).
15 Fischer, C.; Schiavi, R.C.; Edwards, A., et al.: Archs gen. Psychiat. *36*: 431 (1979).

R.S.C. Rodger, Department of Medicine, Royal Victoria Infirmary, Newcastle upon Tyne NE1 4LP (England)

Contr. Nephrol., vol. 38, pp. 116–118 (Karger, Basel 1984)

Zinc Substitution for Male Dialysis Patients: Positive Effect on Preexisting Hypogonadism?

M. Schäfer, R. Mies, M. Vlaho

Köln, FRG

The intention of this study was to evaluate if parenteral substitution of zinc makes any improvement on primary hypogonadism in male hemodialysis patients. This question arises from the controverse findings reported on in the studies of *Antoniou* et al. [1977], *Campieri* et al. [1979], *Mahajan* et al. [1979], and *Brook* et al. [1980]. *Antoniou* et al. [1977] and *Mahajan* et al. [1979] reported on the positive effect of parenteral and oral treatment with zinc on male patients undergoing intermittent dialysis. This effect referred to the androgen metabolism and gonadotropins as well as on sexual activity in dialysis patients with zinc deficiency. *Campieri* et al. [1979] confirmed their findings. Additionally they reported on a decrease in serum prolactin during zinc therapy. *Brook* et al. [1980] could not confirm these findings.

In a simple random blind study 26 male patients undergoing long-term intermittent hemodialysis were examined. Their plasma levels before therapy showed the following values: zinc $11.89 \pm 1{,}65$ µmol/l, testosterone 429.9 ± 136.5 ng/dl, LH $20{,}8 \pm 16.4$ U/l, FSH 13.7 ± 11.6 U/l, prolactin $994.8 \pm 1{,}816.5$ µU/ml. These findings show alterations like those existing in primary hypogonadism. For comparison 10 healthy males aged 20–40 years were examined. Their mean serum levels were as follows: zinc 14.14 ± 2.2 µmol/l, testosterone 712.8 ± 256.5 ng/dl, LH $6{,}7 \pm 1.6$ U/l, FSH 4.3 ± 1.6 U/l.

For the zinc substitution study the 26 male patients undergoing intermittent dialysis had to meet the following criteria: dialysis 3 times a week, age between 20 and 60 years, no testicular atrophy, no therapy with androgens, bromocriptine or a-methyldopa. The patients were randomly divided into two groups. The patients of group B were treated with $61{,}16$ µmol zinc/l of dialysis fluid, while the patients in group A received placebo. Zinc was substituted for 3 months. Zinc and hormone levels were measured before and 1, 4, 9 and 13 weeks after the beginning of substitution therapy.

Mean values and standard deviations of zinc and hormone levels are presented in table I and II.

Table I. Mean and standard deviation of serum zinc (µmol/l) before and after treatment with zinc (n = 13)

Group:		Weeks after treatment				
		0	1	4	9	13
Untreated	Mean	12.13	12.11	12,34[a]	12.81	12.32
	SD	1.97	1.91	1.5	1.54	1.59
Treated	Mean	11.65	14.86	16.7	18.12[a]	17.02
	SD	1.31	3.04	3.01	4.1	3.47

[a] n = 12.

Table II. Mean and standard deviation of hormones before and after treatment with zinc

Parameter		Group			
		untreated		treated	
		week 0	week 13	week 0	week 13
Testosterone, ng/dl	Mean	392.8	404.4	461.1	478.2
	SD	111.9	178.5	154.2	167.1
LH, U/l	Mean	17.5	19.0	24.2	26.9
	SD	8.2	7.8	21.6	27.5
FSH, U/l	Mean	12.9	12.9	14.6	15.4
	SD	9.0	8.2	14.0	13.7
Prolactin, µU/ml	Mean	1,183.5	782.5	806.2	926.9
	SD	2,433.8	1,186.8	934.8	1,150.2

n = 13 in both groups.

(a) The mean serum values of zinc as well as of testosterone, LH and FSH in normal subjects corresponded to the mean values published in the literature.

(b) Comparing normal subjects and the patients of this study, the mean value of serum zinc was significantly lower in dialysis patients. Before the beginning of substitution therapy with zinc there was no difference concerning serum zinc levels between the treated and the untreated group.

(c) The comparison of hormone levels in normal volunteers and dialysis patients before therapy shows that the mean testosterone level was significantly lower in dialysis patients while the plasma levels for LH and FSH were significantly higher. The mean value of serum prolactin was also much higher in the dialysis group. Before therapy there was no difference between the treated and the untreated group concerning the parameters zinc, testosterone, LH, FSH and prolactin.

(d) After 1 week of treatment with zinc the mean level of serum zinc had increased significantly in the treated group. It continued to increase up to the 9th week, but decreased in the 13th week below the levels found in the 9th week. The zinc-treated dialysis fluids were no longer used 2 days before the final measurement.

(e) The changes found in the mean testosterone levels of the treatment group in the course of the study were within physiological limits. The same can be said for the mean values concerning serum levels of LH, FSH and prolactin. Within the untreated group there was no significant change concerning the measured parameters zinc, testosterone, LH, FSH and prolactin.

From the present results the following conclusions can be drawn: In contrast to normal subjects serum zinc and plasma testosterone are lower in most dialysis patients. Concentrations of LH, FSH and prolactin are higher in dialysis patients than in normal controls. Treating dialysis patients parenterally with zinc leads to a significant increase in mean serum zinc concentration. A change in the hormone levels of testosterone, LH, FSH and prolactin could not be achieved. The findings in this study are in agreement with those of *Brook* et al. [1980]. They are not in accordance with those of *Antoniou* et al. [1977], *Campieri* et al. [1979] and *Mahajan* et al. [1979, 1980].

References

Antoniou, L.D.; et al.: Lancet *ii*: 895 (1977).
Antoniou, L.D.; et al.: Lancet *8*: 1034 (1980).
Brook, A.C.; et al.: Lancet *8195*: 618 (1980).
Campieri, C.; et al.: Proc. EDTA *16*: 661 (1979).
Mahajan, S.K.; et al.: Proc. Dialysis Transplant. Forum *9*: 260 (1970).
Mahajan, S.K.; et al.: Trans. Am. Soc. artif. internal Organs *26*: 139 (1980).

Dr. M. Schäfer, Im Falkenhorst 12, D-5000 Köln 90 (FRG)

Contr. Nephrol., vol. 38, pp. 119–125 (Karger, Basel 1984)

Zinc and Sexual Dysfunction

K.B.G. Sprenger[a], J. Schmitz[a], D. Hetzel[b], D. Bundschu[a],
H.E. Franz[a]

[a]Section of Nephrology, Department of Medicine I, and [b]Department of
Internal Medicine I, University of Ulm, FRG

Introduction

In recent years, five studies on the therapeutical effect of zinc on sexual dysfunction in dialysis patients were published, with controversial results [1, 3, 4, 13, 20]. Therefore, we decided to undertake another study on this subject. In the following we will present some essential results.

Methods and Patients

Design of Study

In order to achieve an intraindividual comparison of the therapeutical and placebo effects, the study was performed as a double-blind crossover experiment. The basic measurements were made in a 4-week prephase followed by placebo phase in group A and the therapy phase in group B, each with a duration of 12 weeks. The therapy phase was preceded by a buildup time of 12 weeks for a slow establishment of the therapeutical plasma zinc level. The therapy phase was again followed by an interval of 6 weeks in order to avoid a carryover effect. During this time the plasma zinc level dropped to the initial values. These were followed by a phase of 4 weeks (postphase) during which the final examination was performed.

Zinc Substitution

The therapeutical aim was a plasma zinc concentration between 19.5 and 25 µmol/l according to the data of *Antoniou* et al. [1]. To achieve this, zinc-*L*-hydrogen-aspartate solution was added to 10 liters of commercially available dialysis concentrate as described previously [17].

Patients

At first the male dialysis patients of a center were asked to report on their sexual function. 18 of 33 patients stated that they suffered from sexual dysfunction.

Following a preliminary examination 12 patients remained, consenting to participate in the study after being informed. They were randomized into a placebo and a therapy group.

Protocol of Parameters

Sexual Function

Weekly Investigated Parameters

A diary was kept on libido (8-stage scale), erection (4-stage scale), ejaculation (3-stage scale), sexual activity (4-stage scale), and embrace (4-stage scale) modified according to *Schorsch and Schmidt* [15].

Recordings during Pre- and Postphases

We applied (1) a questionnaire on premorbid, pre-, and postmedication sexual function containing 6 items modified according to *Schorsch and Schmidt* [15]; (2) a questionnaire containing 26 items on sexual attitude [15], and (3) the 'Freiburger Personality Inventory' test for recording of personality differences in the vegetative emotional range containing 212 items [7].

Recordings during the Postphase

A questionnaire with 36 items regarding the therapeutic effect upon sexual function and partner relation was completed [15]. As only 2 of the partners agreed to complete the questionnaires, we had to rely on the patients' information only.

Endocrinological Status

Monthly we investigated testosterone, FSH, LH and prolactin. At the end of placebo and therapy phases an LH-RH test was performed (100 μg i.v.) and semen specimens collected, and during the pre- and postphases the andrological status determined.

Zinc Status and Therapy

At weekly intervals the plasma zinc concentration and monthly the plasma alkaline phosphatase were determined; during the pre-, placebo, therapy, and postphases a taste test was performed.

Blood Sampling, Zinc and Hormonal Determinations, and Taste Quality

Blood sampling and plasma preparation were performed according to the method of *Krivan and Geiger* [12]. All samples were taken after the longest dialysis interval at the same time of the day in a lying position. Plasma and dialysate zinc determinations were performed by flame atomic absorption spectrometry (AAS device model 4000, Perkin Elmer) using the method recently described by *Sprenger and Franz* [16]. Testosterone, LH, FSH, and prolactin were measured by radioimmunology using commercially available kits. In the taste test the detection and recognition threshold for four taste qualities was determined using the 3-drop technique described by *Henkin* et al [9]. The same test solutions were employed in similar concentrations.

Statistical Analysis

The results of 10 patients were evaluated, since 1 of each group had to be excluded due to refusal of the regular controls. Since the results of the single groups did not show any significant differences, the determinations for the combined groups at the end of the placebo and the therapy phase, respectively, were interpreted by Student's paired t test and the nonparametric data by Wilcoxon's paired test.

Results

Hypozincemia was present in all patients. During the prephase and the placebo phase the mean plasma zinc concentrations of 9.6 μmol/l (63 μg/dl) and 9.8 μmol/l (64 μg/dl), respectively, were 19% below the normal limit. During the therapy phase an average dialysate zinc concentration of 26 μmol/l of elementary zinc was required to maintain the plasma zinc concentration in the desired range: mean 23 μmol/l (152 μg/dl).

Hypogeusia improved significantly in all patients. After substitution, the detection and recognition thresholds remained abnormal for the sour taste quality only.

Alkaline phosphatase showed a highly significant increase with zinc substitution, remained constantly in this range, and then decreased again to the initial activity during the decrease phase.

The average *testosterone* level was below the lower normal limit. With a zinc therapy the average testosterone concentration increased slightly in our patients. The marked differences observed in the monthly concentrations are an expression of the known wide physiological range of testosterone values and are not due to technical reasons. The average *LH* level showed a basal increase in our study. A 41% decrease in the LH level occurred during the therapy phase. However, it was not significant in comparison to the placebo phase.

The *FSH* concentration in our patients averaged the normal range and did not significantly decrease under therapy. A *LH-RH test* performed in our patients before and after zinc therapy showed a constant reduced ability of stimulation of the pituitary LH and FSH secretion in both cases.

The average *prolactin* level was slightly increased and did not change significantly under therapy.

Semen specimens were obtained from all patients, usually showing marked oligospermia and motility disturbance. Both did not improve significantly with the zinc substitution.

In all patients sexual dysfunction started after the onset of renal insufficiency. 7 patients were married, 6 had children. Orchidometry was performed before and after zinc therapy. Testicular volumes were found to be in the normal range. 9 patients suffered from erectile disturbances which had lead to an erectile impotence in 4 patients. During the placebo phase, there was an improvement in 3, during the therapy phase in further 2 patients (more than 0.5 points; premorbid number of points: 3.0). A significant difference between these two phases could not be demonstrated.

The ejaculation frequency was markedly diminished in 9 and had recently stopped completely in 5 patients. The administration of a placebo increased the frequency in 3, the administration of zinc in a further 2 patients (more than 0.5 points; premorbid number of points: 2.0). the frequency increase was statistically significant in comparison to the placebo phase ($p < 0.05$).

Accordingly, in 9 patients the frequency of sexual activity (coitus or masturbation, respectively) was in average reduced to approximately one fifth of normal persons of the same age.

During the placebo phase it increased markedly in 2, during the therapy phase in 4 patients (more than 1.0; normal frequency: $1-2$ times per week). The difference between the phases was not statistically significant.

The improvement of the libido after the zinc substitution in comparison to the placebo phase was also not statistically significant. Since the onset of chronic renal insufficiency it had substantially deteriorated in 9 patients. With the therapy it increased markedly (more than 1.0; premorbid number of points: 4.0) in 3 patients and in 4 patients after the placebo phase.

The relation with the female partner − tenderness serving as a control parameter for psychical variations − was in average constant during the entire study.

Discussion

Our patients suffered from a sexual and gonadal dysfunction. In spite of several publications on the endocrine impairments in dialysis patients, it is still unclear whether these are also the cause of sexual dysfunction present in these patients. In most studies the correlation between sexual and gonadal dysfunction was not investigated. Our team as well as other groups [8] found no relation between degree of sexual dysfunction and abnormal hormone levels.

Antoniou et al. [1] were also unable to demonstrate a correlation between testosterone levels and sexual potency. It is, however, known that the metabolic clearance rate of testosterone is elevated in dialysis patients [18]. Furthermore, marked physical and psychical stress may cause a reduction in the testosterone level as well as in spermiogenesis [2, 5, 11, 19, 21]. An elevation of the LH levels could – at least in some of the dialysis patients – also be caused by the reduced metabolic clearance rate of LH [10] and the delayed inactivation of the LH-releasing hormone [6].

In our study it became evident that the sexual function deteriorated markedly during the zinc therapy phase in the patient with the highest increase of testosterone level, whereas in the 3 patients with a constant or decreased testosterone level, it improved clearly.

In the other studies it was not outlined when a symptom was considered to have improved, nor was a definition of the responders given. The control of sexual function was usually determined before and after zinc therapy. With this procedure the therapeutical success in the patients could be retrospectively overestimated. A comparison of the results of the diary and a follow-up questioning showed a clear therapeutical success in 2 of our patients which was, however, not confirmed by the evaluation of the daily recordings.

Antoniou et al. [1] and *Campieri* et al. [4] found an improvement of the sexual function in all patients; *Mahajan* et al. [13] in 9 of 10 patients. *Zetin and Stone* [20] did not observe any improvement in the sexual function of his patients. *Brook* et al. [3] observed an increase in the libido after zinc therapy in 1 patient and an increase in the sexual activity in 2 patients of the placebo group. *Antoniou* et al. [1] and *Mahajan* et al. [13] observed no placebo effect in their patients.

On the average, approximately one third of each patient group will react upon a placebo [14]. In the study by *Antoniou* et al. [1] this is partly explained by the fact that 2 patients of the control group refused the addition of the placebo to the dialysate.

Hypozincemia, hypogeusia with a normalization after zinc substitution and an increase in the alkaline phosphatase activity under zinc administration permit the conclusion that at least a marginal zinc deficiency had existed in our patients.

However, other studies could not prove a state of zinc deficiency. In the studies by *Brook* et al. [3] and *Zetin and Stone* [20] the zinc level was already in the lower normal range before the therapy was started. Therefore, it is not surprising that the patients studied by *Zetin and Stone* [20] showed no subjective improvement of the taste sensation after the zinc therapy. However, it seems that previously no marked hypogeusia peristed, since the patients rated their sensation of taste to be average to good. An objective taste test was not performed. None of the authors controlled the course of other parameters in zinc deficiency.

The dialysate zinc concentration had to be increased to the fourfold dosage used by *Antoniou* et al. [1] in order to achieve a comparable increase in the plasma zinc concentration. It is remarkable that with the same dialysate zinc concentration as used by *Antoniou* et al. [1], *Brook* et al. [3] observed an increase in the plasma zinc concentration by only 17%, whereas in the study by *Zetin and Stone* [20] it even decreased by 8%.

Conclusion

We were not able to show a significant improvement of sexual dysfunction after zinc therapy in a double-blind study. The controversial results of other studies so far are most probably caused by inadequate methods and differences between the patient groups.

References

1   Antoniou, L.D.; Shalhoub, R.J.; Sudhakar, T.; Smith, J.C.: Reversal of uraemic impotence by zinc. Lancet *ii*: 895–898 (1977).
2   Aono, T.; Kurachi, K.; Mizutani, S.; Hamanaka, Y.; Uozumi, T.; Nakasima, T.; Koshiyama, K.; Matsumoto, K.: Influence of major surgical stress on plasma levels of testosterone, luteinizing hormone and follicle stimulating hormone in male patients. J. clin. Endocr. Metab. *35*: 535–542 (1972).
3   Brook, A.C.; Johnston, D.G.; Ward, M.K.; Watson, M.J.; Cook, D.B.; Kerr, D.N.S.: Absence of a therapeutic effect of zinc in the sexual dysfunction of haemodialysed patients. Lancet *ii*: 618–619 (1980).

4 Campieri, C.; Dardeff, A.B.; Borgnino, L.C.; Prandini, R.; Orsoni, G.; Stefoni, S.: Prolactin, zinc and sexual activity in dialysis patients. Proc. EDTA *16*: 661–662 (1979).

5 Charters, A.C.; Odell, W.D.; Thompson, J.C.: Anterior pituitary function during surgical stress and convalescence. Radioimmunoassay measurements of blood TSH, LH, FSH and growth hormone. J. clin. Endocr. Metab. *29*: 63–71 (1969).

6 Destiller, L.A.; Morley, J.E.; Sagel, J.; Pokroy, M.; Rabkin, R.: Pituitary-gonadal function in chronic renal failure: the effect of luteinizing hormone releasing hormone and the influence of dialysis. Metabolism *24*: 711–720 (1975).

7 Fahrenberg, J.; Selg, H.; Hampel, R.: Das Freiburger Persönlichkeitsinventar FPI (Hogrefe, Göttingen 1973).

8 Hagen, C.; Ølgaard, K.; McNeilly, A.S.; Fisher, R.: Prolactin and the pituitary-gonadal axis in male uremic patients on regular dialysis. Acta endocr. Copenh. *82*: 29–38 (1976).

9 Henkin, R.J.; Gill, J.R.; Bartter, F.C.: Studies on thresholds in normal man and patients with adrenal cortical insufficiency: the effect of adrenocorticosteroids. J. clin. Invest. *42*: 727–735 (1963).

10 Holdsworth, S.; Atkins, R.C.; De Kretser, D.M.: The pituitary-testicular axis in men with chronic renal failure. New Engl. J. Med. *269*: 1245–1249 (1977).

11 Kreuz, L.E.; Rose, R.M.; Jennings, R.: Suppression of plasma testosterone levels and psychological stress. Archs. gen. Psychiat. *26*: 479–482 (1972).

12 Krivan, V.; Geiger, H.: Bestimmung von Fe, Co, Cu, Zn, Se, Rb und Cs in NBS-Ochsenleber, Blutplasma und Erythrozyten durch INAA und AAS. Z. analyt. Chem. *305*: 399–404 (1981).

13 Mahajan, S.K. Abbasi, A.A.; Prasad, A.S.; Rabbani, P.; Briggs, W.A.; McDonald, F.D.: Effect of oral zinc therapy on gonadal function in hemodialysis patients A double-blind study. Ann. intern. Med. *97*: 357–361 (1982).

14 Sachs, L.: Angewandte Statistik (Springer, Berlin 1978).

15 Schorsch, E.; Schmidt, G.: Ergebnisse zur Sexualforschung (Wissenschafts-Verlag, Köln 1975).

16 Sprenger, K.B.G.; Franz, H.E.: Viscosity adaption for an automated micro method of flame-AAS and intracellular trace element analysis using pressure decomposition Zinc determination in plasma and erythrocytes. Clin. Chem. *29*: 1522–1526 (1983).

17 Sprenger, K.B.G.; Bundschu, D.; Lewis, K.; Spohn,B.; Schmitz, J.; Franz, H.E.: Improvement of uremic neuropathy and hypogeusia by dialysate zinc substitution: a double blind study. Kidney int. *24(S16)*: 313–317 (1983).

18 Van Kammen, E.; Thijssen, J.H.H.; Schwarz, F.: Sex hormones in male patients with chronic renal failure. 1. The production of testosterone and of androstenedione. Clin. Endocr. *8*: 7–14 (1978).

19 Walker, H.E.: Psychiatric aspects of infertility. Urol. clins. N. Am. *5*: 481–488 (1978).

20 Zetin, M.; Stone, R.A.: Effects of zinc in chronic hemodialysis. Clin. Nephrol. *13*: 20–25 (1980).

21 Zubirám, S.; Goméz-Mont, F.: Endocrine disturbances in chronic human malnutrition. Vitams. Horm. *11*: 97–132 (1953).

Dr. K.B.G. Sprenger, Department of Internal Medicine I, Section of Nephrology, Steinhövelstrasse 9, D-7900 Ulm (FRG)

Contr. Nephrol., vol. 38, pp. 126–128 (Karger, Basel 1984)

Discussion: Zinc Metabolism

There is no question that the many conflicting reports with respect to the action of zinc supplementation in dialysis patients on sexual dysfunction, ageusia, leucocyte or immunological functions, nerve conduction velocity, etc., provided all the elements for a provocative and controversial discussion. It would be unfair, however, not to convey in this summary the strong scepticism of the majority of the panelists. Suspicion prevailed that zinc might ultimately turn out to be a 'red herring'.

In science there is no controversy on issues when items can be measured objectively and analysed quantitatively. Controversies arise when objectively measurable indices are not available or when data are susceptible to subjective interpretation. The latter applies to the assessment of the metabolically reactive zinc pool.

It came as no surprise that the discussion first focused on whether or not low plasma zinc levels in uremic patients indicate the presence of zinc deficiency. Low plasma zinc levels, as found in a variable proportion of dialysed patients, may be induced by factors other than zinc depletion, in particular by acute phase reaction or by malnutrition. Acute phase reaction causes a variety of trace metal abnormalities including hypozincaemia, and this is mediated by induction of hepatic and extrahepatic synthesis of the metal-binding protein metallothionin.

Although tissue zinc levels in various organs of uraemic patients were found to be normal or even increased, this does not rigorously exclude diminution of zinc in a small metabolically active pool. How such depletion of a metabolically active pool could conceivably be brought about was another topic of controversy. Amongst the possibilities touched upon were redistribution of zinc into bone, loss of zinc-containing leucocytes during the dialysis procedure, etc. Clearly, there is a great dearth of, and need for, quantitative data on the metabolically active zinc pool or biochemical indicators thereof in dialysis patients.

Zinc deficiency is most likely to manifest itself when zinc demands are high as, for example, in fetal and postfetal development. Experimentally, zinc deficiency causes teratogenesis or T cell deficiency syndromes in the newborn and delayed puberty in children. The important point was made that neither are birth defects and immunoincompetence syndromes encountered in children born to women on dialysis nor is puberty grossly abnormal in dialysed children. These observations constitute strong arguments against tissue zinc deficiency in uraemia.

The discussion then turned to the action of zinc on gonadal dysfunction. Questions arose as to the rationale of zinc administration and the striking discrepancies between the results of clinical studies on zinc supplementation. The rationale goes back to the observation that zinc concentrations in the gonads are high and that acquired hypogonadism and testicular atrophy are observed in experimental zinc deficiency. Since many enzymes of DNS metabolism and transcription are zinc metalloenzymes, the dependence of spermatogenesis on zinc status is not unexpected. The evidence for the dependence of Leydig cells on zinc is much less clear cut. Even if this tenet is accepted, it is hazardous to conclude that sexual function is a direct reflection of circulating testosterone levels, since human sexual function can often be dissociated from circulating testosterone concentrations. For example, post-pubertal castration does not necessarily eliminate the possibility of having a sex life. The reports of positive effects of zinc supplementation on sexual function (i.e. serum testosterone, LH levels, sperm counts and sexual activity) could only be partially confirmed by the studies of *Sprenger* from Ulm [this issue]and were not confirmed at all by *Rodger* et al. [this issue] from Newcastle, *Schäfer* et al. [this issue] from Cologne and *Massry* from Los Angeles [unpubl. data mentioned during the discussion]. To explain such differences, *Mahajan* pointed out the critical importance of the study duration, as in normal human beings with zinc depletion reversal of sexual abnormalities during repletion required several months. In addition, possible artefacts in the measurement of steroids due to circadian changes, body position and assay specificity were mentioned. Another possible artefact may arise from the fact that with increasing duration of dialysis, sexual function tends to improve in well-dialysed patients up to 2 years after initiation of dialysis.

The question had to be addressed whether on the basis of the information available zinc supplementation should be recommended in dialysis patients in general or at least in dialysis patients which documented hypozincaemia. It was argued, but not universally agreed upon, that zinc supplementation may carry hazards of its own. Experimentally, zinc loading has been shown to cause abnormalities of other trace metals, e.g. decreased coeroloplasmin levels and copper deficiency anaemia, presumably resulting from competition for the trace-element-binding protein metallothionin. In addition, zinc was shown to inhibit lysgloxidase, a key enzyme in collagen biosynthesis. Given the uncertainty of whether dialysis patients derive clinically relevant benefits from zinc supplementation, the majority of panelists felt that zinc, if administered at all, should be given only in controlled clinical studies.

Prof. *E. Ritz*
Dr. *J. Bommer, Heidelberg*

Iron Metabolism

Contr. Nephrol., vol. 38, pp. 129–134 (Karger, Basel 1984)

Iron Kinetics in Healthy Individuals and in Chronic Renal Insufficiency

Joseph W. Eschbach

Department of Medicine, University of Washington, Seattle, Wash., USA

During the past 40 years, isotopes of iron have evolved from experimental use to the quantitation of erythropoiesis, although refinements in the techniques of ferrokinetics continue because various refluxes and the behavior of the transferrin molecule complicate plasma iron exchange [1–3]. This article will review briefly the nature and measurement of internal iron exchange and the changes which occur in chronic renal insufficiency.

Figure 1 details the format of internal iron exchange. All of the iron supplying the tissues passes through plasma as transferrin-bound iron. In the normal individual (NI) about 80% of transferrin-bound iron is taken up by the erythroid marrow and converted within minutes into hemoglobin. After a delay period of about 36 h while the reticulocyte matures, radioiron appears in the circulation and within 2 weeks the newly formed red cells contain about 80% of that injected. In NI about 20% of the iron is wasted by the erythroid marrow which is then processed by the reticuloendothelial cell and either stored or returned to the plasma. The size of the reflux relates to the amount of ineffective erythropoiesis, but is also dependent upon the behavior of the reticuloendothelial cell and the size of its iron stores. With erythroid hyperplasia, little radioiron remains in the reticuloendothelial cell, whereas with inflammation or red cell aplasia, storage is increased. The alternate pathway for radioiron uptake other than the marrow is by the hepatocyte, and its retention of iron appears to directly correlate with plasma iron concentration or transferrin saturation. A third reflux pathway is the extravascular movement of transferrin-bound iron, some of which returns to the plasma and some of which is taken up by various body tissues.

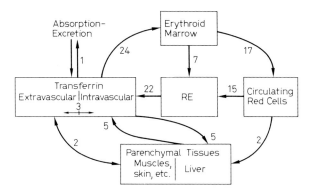

Fig. 1. The amounts of iron (mg/day) exchanging between different body compartments in a 70-kg subject. These data are largely based on ferrokinetic analysis. RE = Reticuloendothelial cell [from ref. 10].

An additional feature to be superimposed on this format is the interaction between cell membrane receptors for transferrin-bound iron, and the transferrin molecule. It is the number of transferrin iron receptors, particularly the diferric form, which determines the amount of iron taken up by any given tissue [4]. Since the amount of diferric transferrin increases proportionately as the transferrin saturation increases, the amount of iron taken up by all tissues progressively increases as transferrin saturation increases.

These concepts of internal iron kinetics have been used to quantitate erythropoiesis. The injection of transferrin-bound radioiron into the circulating blood (at the same transferrin saturation as that of the patient) determines the rate of iron turnover in the plasma (PIT) [1]. The essential measurements are the disappearance rate of radioiron and the plasma iron concentration, and are expressed as:

$$\text{PIT (mg/dl whole blood/day)} = \frac{\text{PI (μg/dl) X plasmatocrit}}{\text{plasma radioiron T}_{1/2}\text{ disappearance (min)}}$$

However, this must be corrected for the effect of plasma iron concentration:

$$\text{Corrected PIT (μg/dl whole blood/day)} = \text{PIT} - \text{PI(μg/dl)} \times 0.0035 \times \text{plasmatocrit [2]}$$

This correction assumes that the patient's plasma iron supply is normal (to saturate receptors) and that reflux is corrected by the factor 0.0035. In NI this direct tissue uptake is 0.50 mg iron/dl whole blood/day. The propor-

Table I. Erythropoiesis in normal subjects, uremia and on RDT

	n	Hct	Tf/m	EIT mg/dl whole blood/day	MTT days
Normal [1]		45	0	0.40	3.3
Phlebotomy-induced anemia [9] (normal plasma iron)		26	0	2.80	1.7
Uremia	7	22	0.6	0.11	3.1
RDT					
Anephric	11	21	1.3	0.28	3.3
Iron excess	13	21	3.4	0.20	3.2
Iron-deficient	36	26	0	0.64	2.5
Peritoneal dialysis	8	24	0.8	0.40	2.9
Hct < 20	30	17	1.0	0.24	3.0
Hct > 30	18	34	0	0.58	2.5

tion of iron coming from the erythroid marrow is the amount of red cell radioactivity found at 10–14 days, provided there is no increase in trapping of iron in the reticuloendothelial cell due to ineffective erythropoiesis. Total effective erythropoiesis is then determined by the formula:

Erythrocyte iron turnover (EIT) (mg/dl whole blood/day) = corrected PIT × red cell activity (%)

This is a simplification of iron kinetics but is reproducible and has provided useful information concerning erythropoiesis in renal disease, primarily because in uncomplicated renal disease, erythropoiesis is effective [5].

The marrow transit time (MTT) indicates the rate of release of marrow reticulocytes and is a function of erythropoietin (Ep) stimulation. As long as there is no stromal disease of the marrow or ineffective erythropoiesis, the MTT indicates the degree of Ep stimulation [6]. The MTT is calculated from the half-time disappearance of radioiron from the plasma to the time of reappearance of half of the radioactivity present at 10 days. In NI this varies between 3 and 3.5 days.

As renal function deteriorates a hypoproliferative anemia develops. This is primarily the consequence of decreased renal Ep production. With

Table II. Improvement in erythropoiesis with RDT

	n	Hct	Tf/m	EIT mg/dl whole blood/day	MTT days
Uremia	7	22	0.6	0.11	3.1
After 12 ± 8 months RDT	7	24	0.9	0.38	2.9
Iron excess	7	20	2.9	0.15	3.1
After 26 ± 15 months RDT	7	24	0.6	0.42	2.8
Androgen therapy					
Before	19	19	1.2	0.27	3.1
After	19	22	0.4	0.45	2.8

the development of anemia, there is a reciprocal increase in storage iron. Ferrokinetic measurements reflect both the decrease in erythropoietic response to anemia and the size of iron stores. The disappearance rate of injected transferrin-bound radioiron is usually prolonged. The PIT is usually at a basal level or even increased (if iron stores are increased), but red cell utilization is usually decreased. Thus the EIT is usually subnormal in uremia (table I).

In table I ferrokinetic data are summarized for regular dialysis therapy (RDT) patients having varying degrees of erythropoiesis. Once RDT is initiated, erythropoiesis improves in some but not all patients [5, 7]. However, there remains a wide spectrum of erythropoiesis, since some patients do not improve (table I, Hct < 20, EIT 0.24 mg/100 ml whole blood/day), whereas others (Hct > 30) have an EIT of up to 0.58 mg/100 ml whole blood/day. Most patients have intermediate levels of erythropoiesis with hematocrits in the 20s. However, even those patients with the best erythropoiesis have EIT levels far short of the 3- to 5-fold increase which would be expected in the anemic but otherwise normal individual [9].

In the following patients on RDT with ferrokinetics several observations have been of interest. Even though erythropoiesis is at basal or subnormal levels, it is susceptible to not only stimulation, but further suppression. Iron overload easily develops when erythropoiesis is subnormal (i.e., EIT < 0.4 mg/100 ml whole blood/day) if transfusions are given repeatedly. Improvement in erythropoiesis not only can occur spontaneously with initi-

Table III. Deterioration in erythropoiesis on RDT

	n	Hct	Tf/m	EIT mg/dl whole blood/day	MTT days
Bilateral nephrectomy					
Before	11	26	1.0	0.53	2.5
After	11	21	1.3	0.28	3.3
Hypertransfusion					
Before	9	21	0.8	0.30	3.2
After	9	31	2.7	0.22	3.2

ation of RDT, but can also occur in suppressed patients with iron excess, particularly if transfusions are withheld and/or androgen therapy is employed. As seen in table II iron excess can be corrected because as erythropoiesis increases, transfusion needs decrease and excess iron is gradually lost via hemodialyzer blood losses [5]. Iron deficiency may eventually develop. The improved erythropoiesis is probably from increased Ep production since the MTT, although inappropriately prolonged, did shorten in all instances (tables I, II). Androgens stimulate Ep production in NI and this has also been demonstrated in patients on RDT [8].

On the other hand, erythropoiesis can be further impaired. Bilateral nephrectomy resulted in a decrease in EIT from 0.53 to 0.28 mg iron/100 ml whole blood/day (table III). Raising the hematocrit to a higher level will reduce the rate of erythropoiesis in NI, and this has also been demonstrated in dialyzed patients [7] (table III). Whether repetitive transfusion will prevent the increase in erythropoiesis observed in some patients is unclear. Hyperparathyroidism without osteitis fibrosa has been claimed to have a detrimental effect on erythropoiesis, but this is conjectural since no supporting ferrokinetic data are available.

These studies support the dominant role of Ep deficiency in the anemia of chronic renal insufficiency (although the moderate shortening in red cell life span also contributes). However, erythropoiesis and the severity of the anemia may be modified. Erythropoietic activity can increase with time. But does this represent an increased capacity to generate Ep from renal or nonrenal tissues, or is it that dialysis removes inhibitors of erythropoiesis? Our ferrokinetic data indicate that when erythropoiesis improves, it is via increased Ep stimulation, but it remains to be clarified whether those patients with persistently poor erythropoiesis are suppressed by inhibitors, frequent transfusion or fail to increase Ep production.

References

1   Finch, C.; Deubelbeiss, K.; Cook, J.; Eschbach, J.; Harker, L.; Funk, D.; Marsaglia, G.; Hillman, R.; Slichter, S.; Adamson, J.; Ganzoni, A.; Giblett, E.: Ferrokinetics in man. Medicine 49: 17–53 (1970).

2   Cook, J.; Marsaglia, G.; Eschbach, J.; Funk, D.; Finch, C.: Ferrokinetics: a biological model for plasma iron exchange in man. J. clin. Invest. 49: 197–205 (1970).

3   Finch, C.; Huebers, H.: The detection of iron overload. New Engl. J. Med. 307: 1702–1703 (1983).

4   Rosemund, A.; Gerber, S.; Huebers, H.; Finch, C.: Regulation of iron absorption and storage iron turnover. Blood 56: 30–37 (1980).

5   Eschbach, J.; Funk, D.; Adamson, J.; Kuhn, I.; Scribner, B.; Finch, C.: Erythropoiesis in patients with renal failure undergoing chronic dialysis. New Engl. J. Med. 276: 653–658 (1967).

6   Labardini,J.; Papyannopoulou, T.; Cook, J.; Adamson, J.; Woodson, R.; Eschbach, J.; Hillman, R.; Finch, C.: Marrow radioiron kinetics. Haematologia 7: 301–312 (1973).

7   Eschbach, J.; Adamson, J.; Cook, J.: Disorders of red blood cell production in uremia. Archs intern. Med. 126: 810–815 (1970).

8   Eschbach, J.; Adamson, J.: Improvement in the anemia of chronic renal failure with fluoxymesterone. Ann. intern. Med. 78: 527–532 (1973).

9   Hillman, R.; Henderson, P.: Control of marrow production by the level of iron supply. J. clin. Invest. 48: 454–460 (1969).

10   Bothwell, T.; Charlton, R.; Cook, J.; Finch, C.: Iron metabolism in man (Blackwell, Oxford 1979).

J.W. Eschbach, MD, Department of Medicine, University of Washington, Seattle, WA 98124 (USA)

Contr. Nephrol., vol. 38, pp. 135–140 (Karger, Basel 1984)

Parameters for the Assessment of Iron Metabolism in Chronic Renal Insufficiency

A. Blumberg, H.R. Marti, Ch. Graber

Medizinische Klinik, Kantonsspital Aarau, Schweiz

The main purpose of assessing iron metabolism is to correct iron deficiency aggravating the anemia of chronic renal failure on the one hand, and if possible to avoid iron overload on the other.

This presentation will concentrate on bone marrow iron stores, iron absorption and serum ferritin concentrations, which will be discussed in relation to chronic renal failure on conservative treatment, on hemodialysis, intermittent and continuous ambulatory peritoneal dialysis, and after transplantation. Other parameters such as serum iron but also transferrin and transferrin saturation have repeatedly been shown to correlate less well with iron status and to be of limited value in chronic renal failure [1–4].

The stainable bone marrow iron is considered the most reliable guide to iron status and will remain the reference method [5]. However, marrow aspiration is not practical as a routine procdure. Gastrointestinal iron absorption is mainly dependent on iron requirements, increasing with diminishing iron stores [6]; it will be of interest to review this relation in chronic renal failure, but obviously the measurement of iron absorption is not suitable for routine use. Finally, the value of serum ferritin will be discussed as it has been found to correlate well with mobilizable iron stores in normal subjects [7].

In patients with chronic renal failure on conservative treatment, increased gastrointestinal blood losses have been demonstrated by *Koch* et al. [8]. At the same time, reduced bone marrow iron was found in almost half the patients. Accordingly, iron absorption, as measured by whole-body counting, has repeatedly been found to be elevated in this group of patients [9–11]. As far as serum ferritin is concerned, only few patients on

Table I. Estimations of iron losses according to various methods

Reference	Measurement of iron loss	Dialyzer	Iron requirements
Edwards et al. [12]	marrow iron	Kiil	2
Hocken and Marwah [13]	hemolysis (dialyzer), counting of blood specimens	Kiil	0.5
Koch et al. [14]	^{51}Cr, whole-body counter	Kiil	2.13
Longnecker et al. [15]	hemolysis (dismantled dialyzer, gauze), counting of specimens	Kiil	2.1 (7.8 liters blood)
Möhring et al. [16]	^{111}In labeling	Gambro Hoeltzenbein	1−2 (3.9−7.2 liters blood)
Present study	Fe therapy according to ferritin	Gambro Hoeltzenbein	1.14 (3.8 liters blood)

conservative treatment have been studied. The sparse results seem to indicate that serum ferritin is a valuable measure of iron status, values below approximately 100 ng/ml being compatible with iron deficiency [10, 11]. If necessary, iron can be given orally to these patients. However, most of the patients we see have been on oral iron for long periods of time (in the hope of improving their anemia) and are not iron deficient.

In hemodialysis patients, the assessment of iron status is of particular importance, since repeated blood losses are inevitable under this condition. Estimations of these losses have varied widely depending on the method of measurement as well as on the method of dialysis (table I). Most studies utilizing Kiil dialyzers have come up with figures around 2 g of iron lost per year [12−15]. With modern dialyzers (such as the Gambro or Hoeltzenbein dialyzer) the calculated figures are somewhat lower, i.e. average losses due to puncture, the dialyzer with lines and blood sampling amount to 6.5−18 ml of blood per dialysis [15, 16]. To this, gastrointestinal losses must be added, so that the total yearly loss still amounts to between 4 and 7 liters of blood. We have tried to evaluate losses by assessing the intravenous iron replacement therapy given whenever serum ferritin fell below 100 ng/ml. In 17 patients followed for 2 years, we found a mean iron loss of 1.14 g/year. With a mean hematocrit of 27%, this corresponds to 3.8 liters of blood, which is in good arrangement with the lower figure of the above-mentioned range. Studies on iron absorption in hemodialyzed patients have yielded somewhat conflicting results. Some groups, including ourselves, found a lowered absorption [1, 17], but this may have been due to insufficient twice-weekly dialysis. In a majority of patients, iron absorption was found to behave normally, increasing with diminishing iron stores [4, 11, 18, 19]. Marrow iron itself is generally regarded as a good measure of body iron stores in hemodialyzed patients [2, 10, 12], only one paper claiming that marrow iron may not be representative of body iron stores [20]. In order to avoid both iron deficiency and iron overload in hemodialysis patients, it was necessary to dispose of a noninvasive and easily repeatable method. During the last years, many groups have shown that serum ferritin concentrations correlate well with bone marrow iron and provide a reliable guide for monitoring iron status and replacement therapy in this group of patients [19, 21–23]. Most results indicate that ferritin levels below 80–100 ng/ml are already compatible with diminished iron stores. Sequential determinations of serum ferritin have become the most useful parameter in assessing the iron status of hemodialyzed patients; in our hemodialyzed patients, routine ferritin determinations are done every 2 months.

Whether replacement therapy should be by the oral or parenteral route is a matter of opinion. Oral replacement is certainly more physiological and is efficient in many patients [18, 24, 25]. In the English literature, it has generally been accepted that antacids impair iron absorption [26]. This fact is surprising because it is based on an abstract describing only 5 persons 4 of whom did not have renal disease. In a study of our own, we could find no influence of antacids in 6 hemodialyzed patients in whom iron absorption with and without aluminium-containing antacids was measured by whole-body counting [27] (fig. 1). Nevertheless, oral replacement therapy may be uncertain due to the large number of medications ingested by hemodialyzed patients. *Anderson* et al. [28], for instance, found a mean of 7.7 medications prescribed per patient. In our own patients, the figure was 4.3 which is still rather high. Therefore one can argue that intravenous iron may be necessary in patients who do not respond satisfactorily to oral iron or in those who seem to be unreliable.

In patients on intermittent peritoneal dialysis, iron absorption and serum ferritin seem to behave normally, but only few data are available. For patients on continuous ambulatory peritoneal dialysis, no data could be found. For this reason, we compared serum ferritin concentrations with bone marrow iron stores in 20 patients on continuous ambulatory

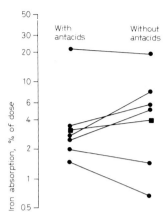

Fig. 1. Iron absorption (as measured by whole-body counter) with and without aluminium hydroxide in 6 patients on maintenance hemodialysis [from ref. 27].

peritoneal dialysis. We found a good correlation between the two parameters with a correlation coefficient of 0.84. Again, values below approximately 80 ng/ml were a good indicator of iron deficiency. In these patients, who are on slightly less medication than hemodialyzed patients (3.6 v. 4.3 in our experience) and who need lesser amounts of iron, oral supplementation seems to be logical.

In transplanted patients, finally, only a limited amount of information is available. Absorption has been described as normal in a fairly recent study [29]. Serum ferritin is in the usual range [23], but, to the best of our knowledge, the relation of ferritin to marrow iron has not been studied as yet. Based on anecdotal observations one would suspect that serum ferritin is a valuable parameter of iron status in this group as well.

The presented data can be summarized as follows:

(1) The assessment of bone marrow iron stores remains the reference method but is not suitable for repeated routine use.

(2) Iron absorption is normal in chronic renal failure.

(3) Serum ferritin correlates well with bone marrow iron stores in chronic renal failure.

(4) Serum ferritin is the most useful parameter for the clinical assessment of iron metabolism in chronic renal failure, especially so in hemodialyzed patients who are at risk of derangements.

References

1   Blumberg, A.; Chappuis, C.: Die enterale Eisenresorption bei der chronischen Niereninsuffizienz unter Langzeitdialyse-Behandlung. Klin. Wschr. *49*: 41 (1971).

2   Bell, J.D.; Kincaid, W.R.; Morgan, R.G.; Bunce, H.; Alpertin, J.B.; Sarles, H.E.; Remmers, A.R., Jr.: Serum ferritin assay and bone-marrow iron stores in patients on maintenance hemodialysis. Kidney int. *17*: 237 (1980).

3   Craswell, P.; Hunt, F.; Davies, L.; Russo, A.; Goethart, J.; Halliday, J.: Serum ferritin as an index of body iron stores in patients on chronic haemodialysis. Aust. N.Z. J. Med. *8*: 38 (1978).

4   Milman, N.; Larson, L.: Iron absorption in patients with chronic uremia undergoing regular hemodialysis. Acta med. scand. *199*: 193 (1976).

5   Weinfeld, A.: Iron stores; in Hallberg, Hartwert, Vanotti, Iron deficiency, p. 329 (Academic Press, London 1970).

6   Pirzio-Biroli, G.; Finch, C.A.: Iron absorption. III. The influence of iron stores on iron absorption in the normal subject. J. Lab. clin. Med. *55*: 216 (1960).

7   Jacobs, A.; Warwood, M.: Ferritin in serum. New Engl. J. Med. *292*: 951 (1975).

8   Koch, K.M.; Bechstein, P.B.; Fassbinder, W.; Kaltwasser, P.; Schoeppe, W.; Werner, E.: Occult blood loss and iron balance in chronic renal failure. Proc. Eur. Dial. Transplant. Ass. *12*: 362 (1976).

9   Sulin. A.W.; Blumberg, A.: Die enterale Eisenresorption bei Patienten mit chronischen Nierenkrankheiten. Schweiz. med. Wschr. *101*: 883 (1971).

10 Milman, N.; Christensen, T.E.; Strandberg Pedersen, N.; Visfeldt, J.: Serum ferritin and bone marrow iron in non-dialysis, peritoneal dialysis and hemodialysis patients with chronic renal failure. Acta med. scand. *207*: 201 (1980).

11 Milman, N.: Iron absorption measured by whole body counting and relation to marrow iron stores in chronic uremia. Clin. Nephrol. *17*: 77 (1982).

12 Edwards, M.S.: Pegrum, G.D.; Curtis, J.R.: Iron therapy in patients on maintenance haemodialysis. Lancet *ii*: 491 (1970).

13 Hocken, A.G.; Marwah, P.K.: Iatrogenic contribution to anaemia of chronic renal failure. Lancet *i*: 164 (1971).

14 Koch, K.M.; Patyna, W.D.; Shaldon, S.; Werner, E.: Anemia of the regular hemodialysis patient and its treatment. Nephron *12*: 405 (1974).

15 Longnecker, R.E.; Goffinet, J.A.; Hendler, E.D.: Blood loss during maintenance hemodialysis. Trans. Am. Soc. artif. internal Organs *20*: 135 (1974).

16 Möhring, K.; Sinn, H.; Schüler, H.W.; Horsch, R.; Krüger, H.; Asbach, H.W.: Comparative evaluation of iatrogenic sources of blood loss during maintenance dialysis. Proc. Eur. Dial. Transplant. Ass. *13*: 233 (1976).

17 Boddy, K.; Lawson, D.H.; Linton, A.L.; Will, G.: Iron metabolism in patients with chronic renal failure. Clin. Sci. *39*: 115 (1970).

18 Eschbach, J.W.; Cook, J.D.; Finch, C.A.: Iron absorption in chronic renal disease. Clin. Sci. *38*: 191 (1970).

19 Eschbach, J.W.; Cook, J.D.; Scribner, B.H.; Finch, C.A.: Iron balance in hemodialysis patients. Ann. intern. Med. *87*: 710 (1977).

20 Ali, M.; Fayemi, O.; Rigolosi, R.; Frascino, J.; Marsden, T.; Malcolm, D.: Hemosiderosis in hemodialysis patients. J. Am. med. Ass. *244*: 343 (1980).

Serum ferritin assay and iron status in chronic renal failure and haemodialysis. Br. med. J. *i*: 546 (1975).

22   Mirahmadi, K.S.; Paul, W.L.; Winter, R.L.; Dabir-Vaziri, N.; Byer, B.; Gorman, J.T.; Rosen, S.M.: Serum ferritin level. Determinant of iron requirement in hemodialysis patients. J. Am. med. Ass. *237*: 601 (1977).

23   Hofmann, V.; Descoeudres, C.; Montandon, H.; Galeazzi, R.L.; Straub, P.W.: Serumferritin bei Niereninsuffizienz, Hämodialyse und nach Nierentransplantation. Schweiz. med. Wschr. *108*: 1835 (1978).

24   Strickland, I.D.; Chaput de Saintonge, D.M.; Boulton, F.E.; Francis, B.; Roubikova, J.; Waters, J.I.: The therapeutic equivalence of oral and intravenous iron in renal dialysis patients. Clin. Nephrol. *7*: 55 (1977).

25   Heinecke, G.; Finke, K.; Konner, K.; Rath, K.; Schulz, E.: Zur Frage der Wirksamkeit einer oralen Eisensubstitution bei Dauerdialysepatienten. Klin. Wschr. *52*: 979 (1974).

26   Rastogi, S.; Padilla, F.; Boyd, C.M.: Effect of aluminum hydroxide on iron absorption (Abstract) Kidney int. *8*: 417 (1975).

27   Blumberg, A.: Der Einfluss Aluminiumhydroxyd-haltiger Antazida auf die enterale Eisenresorption von Langzeitdialysepatienten. Schweiz. med. Wschr. *107*: 1064 (1977).

28   Anderson, R.J.; Melikian, D.M.; Gambertoglio, J.G.; Berns, A.; Cadnapaphornchai, P.; Eyan, D.J.; Goldberg, J.P.; Heinrich, W.L.; Hicks, D.L.; Kovalchik, M.T.; Olin, D.B.: Prescribing medication in long-term dialysis units. Archs intern. Med. *142*: 1305 (1982).

29   Milman, N.; Larsen, L.: Iron absorption after renal transplantation. Acta med. scand. *200*: 25 (1976).

Dr. A. Blumberg, Medizinische Klinik, Kantonsspital Aarau,
CH-5000 Aarau (Switzerland)

Contr. Nephrol., vol. 38, pp. 141–152 (Karger, Basel 1984)

The Assessment of Iron Stores in Children on Regular Dialysis Treatment

D.E. Müller-Wiefel[a], R. Waldherr[b], D. Feist[a], G. van Kaick[c]

[a]Children's Hospital and [b]Institute of Pathology, University of Heidelberg, and [c]German Cancer Research Center, Heidelberg, FRG

In children on regular dialysis treatment (RDT) various factors influence iron stores (IS). On one hand IS are decreased by an exaggerated *blood loss* of about 15 ml/m^2/day [21] via the gastrointestinal tract, the dialyzer system and blood sampling. Children with uropathies are predestined, because of their increased need for iron, as a result of a relatively better erythropoiesis in contrast to other primary renal diseases [26]. On the other hand IS are exaggerated especially by *blood transfusions*, which to date can hardly be avoided in children on RDT, increased *hemolysis* combined with a decreased *erythropoiesis* [28], or unreflected parenteral *iron treatment*, especially in genetically determined (HLA A3, B7) children [25].

Serum Ferritin

Due to therapeutic consequences, diagnostic parameters assessing IS are of great value for the clinician. The best parameter has to be reliable, suitable and non invasive. Within the last decade an increasing number of authors have urged that serum ferritin (SF) values fulfill these criteria irrespective of the patients' sex and age and the method used (3–5, 12, 13, 15, 17, 18, 20, 22]. In children on RDT the method is also useful insofar as definite consequences can be drawn concerning the need for *oral iron treatment*. When treating 5 children on RDT with normal SF, as determined by an immunoradiometric assay in a heterologous antibody system [27], with oral iron sulfate (5mg/kg) over a mean period of 6 months, there was a further increase of SF, but a concomitant fall of hemoglobin (fig. 1a). In spite of the same mode of treatment in 12 children on RDT with decreased

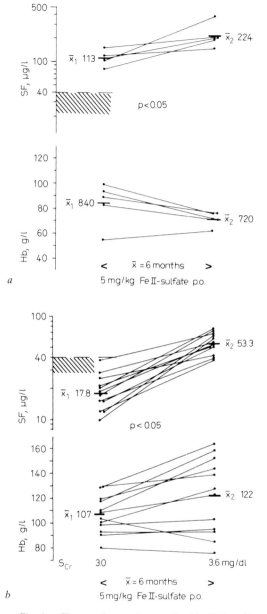

Fig. 1. a Change of normal serum ferritin (SF) and hemoglobin (Hb) concentrations in 5 children on regular hemodialysis treatment (RDT) with mean values (x̄) at start (1) and at the end (2) of oral iron treatment.▨= Range of decreased values. *b.* Change of decreased SF values in 12 children on RDT under the same conditions as in figure 1a.

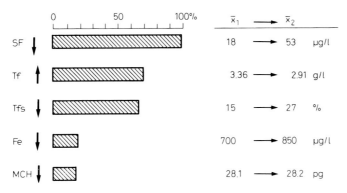

Fig. 2. Comparison of serum ferritin (SF) concentrations of the patients in figure 1b with other parameters of iron deficiency in peripheral blood: serum transferrin (Tf); transferrin saturation (Tfs); serum iron (Fe); mean corpuscular hemoglobin (MCH). Either an increase (↑) or decrease (↓) are indicative of iron deficiency and are given in percent of the number of decreased SF values (= 100%). The changes of the corresponding mean values at start ($\bar{x}_1$) and the end ($\bar{x}_2$) of iron treatment are given on the right side.

SF, the increase of the values was accompanied by an elevation of hemoglobin (fig. 1b). In accordance with the literature on adults, SF can be a helpful parameter not only for *starting* but also for *monitoring* iron treatment [6, 10, 29]. SF seems to be superior to other diagnostic parameters of iron deficiency and peripheral blood such as transferrin, transferrin saturation, serum iron or mean corpuscular hemoglobin, only partially indicating the child's need for iron (fig. 2). These observations are in line with results in adults too [13, 14, 19]. On the other hand it is well known that, in the case of infection or hepatic damage, SF levels become unreliable in reflecting body IS [24]. Therefore we have tried to evaluate the best substituting parameter in the peripheral blood indicating iron deficiency in RDT children.

Other Peripheral Blood Parameters of Iron Deficiency

A significant correlation ($p < 0.001$) could be obtained between SF and serum *transferrin*, however, with a coefficient of correlation of only 0.37. In about 10% of reduced SF, iron deficiency was not indicated (fig. 3a). As documented in previous investigations serum transferrin is a better parameter of nutrition than iron metabolism [23]. The correlation between

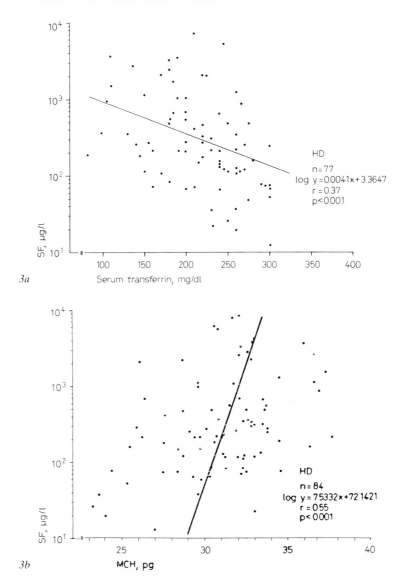

3a

3b

SF and *mean corpuscular hemoglobin* was somewhat better (r = 0.55; fig. 3b). However, decreased mean corpuscular hemoglobin was indicative of iron deficiency in only about 50%. Even better from the statistical point of *view* was the correlation between SF and the *serum iron* level (r = 0.56; fig. 3c); but in no case of decreased SF was the serum iron level reduced.

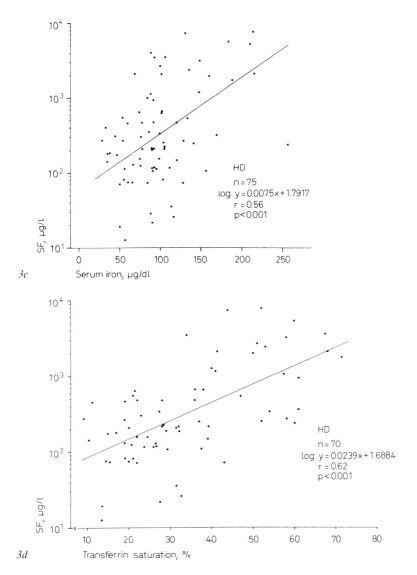

3c

3d

Although the coefficient of correlation between SF and *transferrin satura-tion* was 0.62, reduced transferrin saturation was found three times more often with normal than with decreased IS (fig. 3d). The correlation between SF and mean corpuscular volume was in the same range (r = 0.62). Reduced values, however, indicated iron deficiency in all cases but one

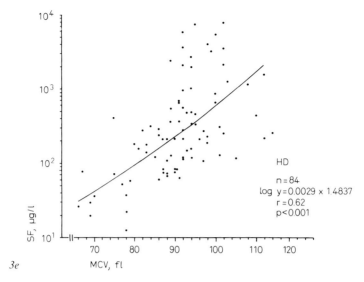

Fig. 3. Correlation of serum ferritin (SF) with serum transferrin(*a*); mean corpuscular hemoglobin (MCH) (*b*); serum iron (*c*); transferrin saturation (*d*), and mean corpuscular volume (MCV) (*e*) in children on regular hemodialysis treatment (HD).

(fig. 3e). In accordance with investigations in adults [14], we therefore propose the mean corpuscular erythrocyte volume to substitute SF levels in the diagnosis of iron deficiency in RDT children with infection or hepatopathy – of course after exclusion of aluminium intoxication. Mean corpuscular volume is unable to indicate increased iron stores.

Other Parameters of Iron Overload

In the case of an unclearly elevated SF, hypersiderosis is said to be best proven by quantitative or semiquantitative *histochemical* iron determination in different tissue specimens [1, 8, 11, 19, 31].

In this context, semiquantitative examination of the *bone marrow* has mostly been favored [5, 8, 19]. Reliable results can only be expected in marrow biopsies, not in smears, taking into consideration intra- and extracellular iron staining. In our small group of marrow-biopsied RDT children, there was no significant correlation ($p > 0.05$) between SF and bone marrow iron (fig. 4). The number of siderin-containing cells per square mil-

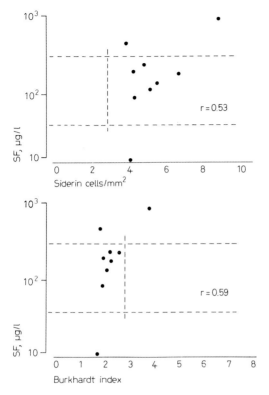

Fig. 4. Correlation of serum ferritin (SF) with bone marrow iron in biopsies of the iliac crest (Yamshidi technique) in 9 children on regular dialysis treatment (RDT). The intracellular iron is expressed by the number of siderin-containing cells per square millimeter, the extracellular one by the *Burkhardt* [8] index.

limeter was above the normal value for adults in all patients, even in 1 child with reduced SF. There was a closer, but nonetheless insignificant correlation between SF and the extracellular iron content as defined by the *Burkhardt* [8] index. An increased index was only found in the 1 child with the highest SF value. On the whole in RDT children the relationship between bone marrow iron and SF remains questionable. Interestingly, disturbances of this correlation have only recently been pointed out in adults with renal failure [1, 2, 16], but have been interpreted as a consequence of parenteral iron therapy, which our children never received.

The organ which seems to represent best total body IS in terminal renal failure is the *liver*. For histochemical diagnosis one has to differen-

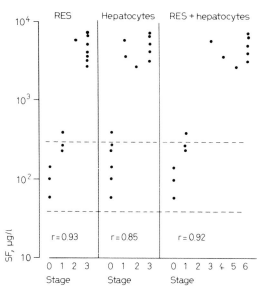

Fig. 5. Correlations of serum ferritin (SF) with liver iron content in biopsy specimens of 14 children on regular hemodialysis treatment (RDT) by Prussian blue staining and staging from 0 to 3+ in the reticulo-endothelial system (RES), the hepatocytes or both cell compartments together, according to [32].

tiate between iron staining of the reticulo-endothelial system (RES), on one hand, and the hepatocytes on the other hand. In contrast to bone marrow, SF correlated significantly with both the RES and hepatocyte iron (p < 0.001; fig. 5). In all cases of SF levels above 2,500 μ /l, RES iron storage was classified by 3+ or 2+ but in 1 child. We conclude that liver IS are more representative of total body IS in RDT children than bone marrow IS are, which is in line with recent publications in adults [1, 2.]. However, the assessment of IS by biopsy is an invasive method which should be restricted to children with pathologic diagnostic liver tests.

Avoiding liver biopsy we preferred examination by *computerized tomography* to estimate tissue iron content by means of its density [9]. To get a reliable integrated mean value only one or two sections are necessary. In 8 RDT children with different degrees of iron overload, there was a significant positive correlation (p < 0.01) between SF and liver density, as expressed by *Hounsfield* units (fig. 6). In all cases increased SF values were accompanied by an increased liver density of above 65 U, which is the upper limit in childhood. Not only because of its non-invasive character but

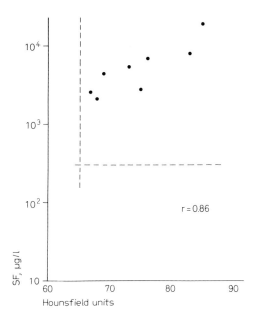

Fig. 6. Correlation of serum ferritin (SF) with computerized liver density in 8 children on regular dialysis treatment (RDT) expressed in Hounsfield units. − − − = Upper limit of both parameters in children.

also because of its accuracy, liver CT should be preferred to tissue biopsy for clarifying elevated SF levels. Magnetic susceptibility measurements of the liver might become an alternative in the future [7].

Conclusive Diagnostic and Therapeutic Procedure

For diagnostic and therapeutic reasons the pediatric-clinical indications for each parameter of IS discussed are summarized conclusively (fig. 7): SF concentration should be measured at 3-month intervals. In the case of reduced SF levels (< 40 µg/l) [27] iron deficiency is proven and oral treatment with iron sulfate is indicated. If the SF level ranges between 40 and 2,000 µg/l, no iron therapy is necessary in the absence of hepatopathy or infection. However, in the presence of one of these conditions a mean corpuscular volume of < 70 fl should favor the start of oral iron treatment. In the case of evident SF elevation above 2.000 µg/l without hepatopathy, liver density has to be measured by computerized tomography, and only with an

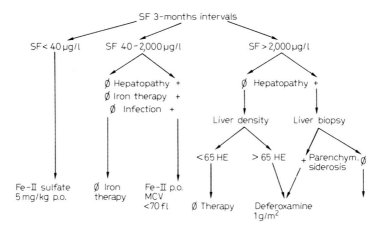

Fig. 7. Diagnostic and therapeutic procedure in regard to the iron status of CRF children.

increased density does an *iron-binding therapy* [30] with deferoxamine seem to be indicated. If pathologic serum parameters of liver function are present, liver biopsy properly gives evidence to prove hypersiderosis and then iron-binding therapy should start. There is no need for bone marrow biopsy for the diagnosis of iron overload.

References

1   Ali, M.; Fayemi, A.O.; Rigolosi, R.; Frascino, J.; Marsden, T.; Malcom, D.: Hemosiderosis in hemodialysis patients: an autopsy study of 50 cases. J. Am. med. Ass. *244*: 343–345 (1980).

2   Ali, M.; Rigolosi, R.; Fayemi, A.O.; Braun, E.V.; Frascino, J.; Singer, R.: Failure of serum ferritin levels to predict bone-marrow iron content after intravenous iron-dextran therapy. Lancet *i*: 652–655 (1982).

3   Aljama, P.; Ward, K.M.; Pierides, A.M.; Eastham, E.J.; Ellis, H.A.; Feest, T.G.; Conceicao, S.; Kerr, D.S.: Serum ferritin concentration, a reliable guide to iron overload in uremic and hemodialysed patients. Clin. Nephrol. *10*: 101 (1978).

4   Beallo, R.; Dallmann, P.R.; Schoenfeld, P.Y.; Humphreys, M.H.: Serum ferritin and iron deficiency in patients on chronic hemodialysis. Trans. Am. Soc. artif. internal Organs *22*: 73 (1976).

5   Bell, J.D.; Kincaid, W.R.; Morgan, R.G.; Bunce, H.; Alperin, J.B.; Sarles, H.E.; Remmers, A.R.: Serum ferritin assay and bone-marrow iron stores in patients on maintenance hemodialysis. Kidney int. *17*: 237 (1980).

6   Birgegard, G.; Nilsson, P.; Wide, L.: Regulation of iron therapy by serum ferritin esti-
     mations in patients on chronic hemodialysis. Scand. J. Urol. Nephrol. *15*: 69–72 (1981).
7   Brittenham, G.M.; Farrell, D.E.; Harris, J.W.; Feldman, E.S.; Danish, E.H.; Muir,
     W.A.; Tripp, J.H.; Bellon, E.M.: Magnetic-susceptibility measurements of human iron
     stores. New Engl. J. Med. *307*: 1671–1674 (1982).
8   Burkhardt, R.: Iron overload of bone-marrow and bone; in: Kief, Iron metabolism and
     its disorders, pp. 264–272 (Excerpta Medica, Amsterdam 1975).
9   Chapman, R.W.G.; Williams, G.; Bydder, G.; Dick, R.; Sherlock, S.; Kreel, L.: Com-
     puted tomography for determining liver iron content in primary hemochromatosis. Brit.
     med. J. *i*: 440–442 (1980).
10   Cotterill, A.M.; Flather, J.N.; Cattell, W.R.; Marnett, M.D.; Baker, L.R.I.: Serum
     ferritin concentration and oral iron treatment in patients on regular hemodialysis. Br.
     med. J *i*: 790–791 (1979).
11   Van Eijk, H.G.; Tio, T.H.; Bos, G.: Iron in skin biopsies. Arch. dermatol. Forsch. *251*:
     245–248 (1975).
12   Ellis, D.: Serum ferritin compared with other indices of iron status in children and teen-
     agers undergoing maintenance hemodialysis. Clin. Chem. *25*: 741–744 (1979).
13   Eschbach, J.W.; Cook, J.D.; Scribner, B.H.; Finch, C.A.: Iron balance in hemodialysis
     patients. Ann. intern. Med. *87*: 710–713 (1977).
14   Gokal, R.; Millard, P.R.; Weatherall, D.J.; Callender, S.T.E.; Ledingham, J.G.G.;
     Oliver, D.O.: Iron metabolism in hemodialysis patients. Q. Jl Med. *48*: 369 (1979).
15   Hussein, S.; Prieto, J.; O'Shea, M.; Hoffland, A.V.; Baillod, R.A.; Moorehead, J.F.:
     Serum ferritin assay and iron status in chronic renal failure and hemodialysis. Br. med.
     J. *i*: 546 (1975).
16   Lynn, K.L.; Mitchell, T.R.; Shepperd, J.: Serum ferritin concentration in patients re-
     ceiving maintenance hemodialysis. Clin. Nephrol. *14*: 124–127 (1980).
17   Marco-Franco, J.E.; Alarcon, A.; Morey, A.; Piza, C.; Bestard, J.; Mairata, S.;
     Galmes, A.; Dalmau, M.: Serum ferritin in hemodialysis. Nephron *32*: 57–59 (1982).
18   Milman, N.; Christensen, T.E.; Pedersen, N.S.; Visfeldt, J.: Serum ferritin and bone
     marrow iron in non-dialysis, peritoneal dialysis and hemodialysis patients with chronic
     renal failure. Acta med. scand. *207*: 201 (1980).
19   Milman, N.; Christensen, T.E.; Visfeldt, J.: Diagnostic efficiency of various laboratory
     tests in the assessment of bone marrow iron stores in patients with chronic uremia.
     Scand. J. Haematol. *26*: 257–264 (1981).
20   Mirahmadi, K.S.; Wellington, L.P.; Wieher, R.L.; Dabir-Vaziri, N.; Byer, B.; Gor-
     man, J.T.; Rosen, S.M.: Serum ferritin level. Determinant of iron requirement in
     hemodialysis patients. J. Am. med. Ass. *238*: 601 (1977).
21   Müller-Wiefel, D.E.; Sinn, H.; Gilli, G.; Schärer, K.: Hemolysis and blood loss in chil-
     dren with chronic renal failure. Clin. Nephrol. *8*: 581–586 (1977).
22   Müller-Wiefel, D.E.; Wolf, E.; Schönberg, D.; Schärer, K.: Serum-ferritin concentra-
     tions in children with chronic renal failure. Proc. Eur. Dial. Transpl. Ass. *15*: 625–627
     (1978).
23   Müller-Wiefel, D.E.; Borm, U.; Palm, F.; Wolf, E.: Proteins of iron metabolism in chil-
     dren with chronic renal failure; in Bulla, Dialysis and kidney transplantation in children,
     pp. 115–127 (Bibliomed, Kassel 1979).
24   Müller-Wiefel, D.E.: Diagnostische Bedeutung des Serumferritins bei renaler Anämie.
     Dt. med. Wschr. *105*: 1096–1097 (1980).

25   Müller-Wiefel, D.E.; Lenhard, V.; Schärer, K.: Body iron stores in children with chronic renal failure in relation to HLA phenotypes. Proc. Eur. Dial. Transpl. Ass. *18*: 524–530 (1981).

26   Müller-Wiefel, D.E.; Querfeld, U.; Mehls, O.; Schärer, K.: Body iron stores in children with chronic renal failure in relation to primary renal disease. Abstracts. 8th Int. Congr. Nephrology, Athens, 1981, p. 345.

27   Müller-Wiefel, D.E.; Brendlein, F.; Ehrlich, J.; Brandeis, W.E.; Schärer, K.: Serumferritin bei Kindern mit Störungen der Eisenbilanz. Helv. paediat. Acta *37*: 245–256 (1982).

28   Müller-Wiefel, D.E.: Renale Anämie im Kindesalter. Untersuchungen zur Pathogenese und Kompensation (Thieme, Stuttgart 1982).

29   Parker, P.A.; Izard, M.W.; Maher, J.F.: Therapy of iron deficiency anemia in patients on maintenance dialysis. Nephron *23*: 181–186 (1979).

30   Simon, P.; Bonn, F.; Guezennec, M.; Tanquerel, T.: La surchage en fer chez les patients hémodialysés: critères diagnostiques, indication et résultats du traitement par desferrioxamine. Néphrologie *2*: 165–170 (1981).

31   Sobolewski, S.; Lawrence, A.C.K.; Bagshaw, P.: Human nails and body iron. J. clin. Path. *31*: 1068–1072 (1978).

32   Scheuer, P.J.; Williams, R.; Muir, A.R.: Hepatic pathology in relatives of patients with hemochromatosis. J. Path. Bact *84*: 53–64 (1962).

Priv.-Doz. Dr. D.E. Müller-Wiefel, Division of Pediatric Nephrology,
University Children's Hospital, Im Neuenheimer Feld 150, D-6900 Heidelberg (FRG)

Contr. Nephrol., vol. 38, pp. 153–166 (Karger, Basel 1984)

Patterns of Iron Storage in Patients with Severe Renal Failure

Frank L. Van de Vyver[a], Arnold O. Vanheule[b], Armand H. Verbueken[a],
Patrick D'Haese[b], Walter J. Visser[c], Arline B. Bekaert[a],
René E. Van Grieken, Norbert Buyssens[a], Willy De Keersmaecker[a],
Walter Van den Bogaert[a], Marc E. De Broe[a]

[a]Departments of Nephrology-Hypertension, Nuclear Medicine, Chemistry and Pathology, University of Antwerp, Wilrijk, Belgium; [b]Department of Toxicology, University of Gent, Belgium; [c]Laboratory of Bone Metabolism, University of Utrecht, The Netherlands

Introduction

It is difficult to determine iron requirements in patients being treated by chronic hemodialysis. Some suffer from iron deficiency due to chronic blood losses [1], while others have increased iron stores due to numerous blood transfusions or intravenous iron therapy [2].

It has been argued that iron therapy in chronic hemodialysis patients is necessary [1], but, recently, the undesirable effects of excessive iron therapy have been demonstrated [3, 4]. Several authors have proposed serum ferritin levels as a reliable guide for iron therapy in chronic hemodialysis patients [5–18].

In this study, we set out to try to answer some questions regarding the iron requirements in patients with severe renal failure:

(1) Is there proportionate iron storage in the different iron storage compartments? (2) What is the ultrastructural localization of stored iron? Is there an ultrastructural relationship between iron and other elements? (3) What is the relationship between serum ferritin levels and the amount of storage iron and iron administration? (4) Are other parameters, such as free erythrocyte protoporphyrin (FEP) levels, more reliable in guiding iron therapy?

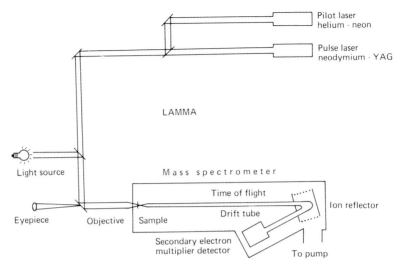

Fig. 1. Schematic representation of the laser microprobe mass spectrometer (LAMMA).

Patients and Methods

81 patients (61 living and 20 deceased), with severe renal failure, were studied for iron storage compartments. The group of living patients consisted of 46 patients being treated by chronic hemodialysis and 15 without dialysis treatment, with serum creatinine levels above 4 mg/dl. 15 of the 20 deceased patients had been treated by chronic hemodialysis. Only 5 of the total patient group had received iron therapy besides blood transfusions.

The bone iron stores were estimated by studying transiliac bone biopsies obtained with a 7 mm diameter trephine (Bordier-Meunier) [19]. Bone marrow smears were stained for iron, and the reticuloendothelial iron was graded from 0 to 6+ [20] by two different observers. The iron content of wet tissue bone marrow specimens was estimated by means of flameless atomic absorption spectrometry (AAS) after destruction with nitric acid. Thus, two parameters were obtained for bone marrow iron: (1) a cytological grading of reticuloendothelial bone marrow iron, and (2) a chemical measurement of bone marrow iron.

In the 20 autopsy patients, liver iron was also investigated. The methods used to study liver iron were the same as those used for bone marrow iron. Thus, three parameters of liver iron storage were obtained: (1) the histologically graded Kupffer-cell iron (graded from 0 to 4+) [21]; (2) the histologically graded hepatocyte iron, the so-called parenchymal liver iron (also graded 0 to 4+) and (3) the chemical measurement of liver iron obtained by means of flameless AAS of wet tissue.

Laser microprobe mass analysis (LAMMA) [22] was used for the study of the ultrastructural localization of bone marrow and liver iron. The LAMMA-500 of Leybold-Heraeus was used (fig. 1). The histological section is viewed with a binocular light microscope. The system is equipped with two lasers. The first is a low-powered (2 mW) red helium-neon laser that can

Table I. Evaluation of the LAMMA technique

Advantages	Disadvantages
Multielemental microanalysis	spatial resolution of analysis (1−3 μm) larger than some cellular organelles
Fast analysis	section thickness 0.1−2 μm
High sensitivity	moderate quality of the light microscopic view
Low detection limits (ppm range) compared to electron probe X-ray microanalysis (several 1,000 ppm)	semiquantitative character
Isotopic information	organic background interference at trace levels
Organic and inorganic molecular information	

be focused to a 1-μm diameter spot to outline the analytical region. Colinear with this search laser is a neodymium-YAG laser that provides a high power pulse that is able to vaporize and ionize a selected area of some square μm of a thin section. The positive or negative ions produced are separated in a time-of-flight mass spectrometer. The separated ions are detected according to their mass producing a complete mass spectrum for each laser pulse.

Table I gives some features of the LAMMA technique. While the light microscopic view is of moderate quality, electron micrographs taken before and after the LAMMA analysis provide more detailed information. Although the mass spectra are not quantitative, the low detection limits offer an important advantage, relative to other micro-analytical procedures. The methyl methacrylate-embedded bone biopsy sections (2 μ thick) of 3 patients with dialysis osteomalacia and high bone aluminum content, were compared with the LAMMA technique. The first two patients also showed an elevated bone iron content relative to the third patient.

In the first patient, a liver biopsy was also examined. The liver biopsy was treated according to routine transmission electron microscopy procedures. Thin 0.2-μm sections were cut on a Reichert ultramicrotome and stained with alcoholic uranyl acetate and lead citrate. The sectioned specimens were directly mounted on copper finder-grids to avoid additional organic mass interferences originating from the carrier foil. Before the LAMMA analyses were performed, transmission electron micrographs were taken of the cellular regions of interest with a Zeiss EM 109 instrument. Another series of transmission electron micrographs taken after the LAMMA analysis provided records of the nature and the amount of evaporated and analyzed subcellular fragments. The image quality of the electron micrographs was not optimal, due to the thickness of the sections necessary for LAMMA analysis. However, we did consider it possible to identify the cellular organelles ultrastructurally.

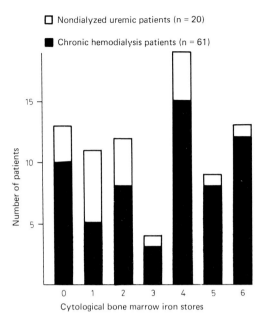

Fig. 2. Distribution of patients with severe renal failure with regard to cytologically graded reticulo endothelial bone marrow iron stores (n = 81).

Patients from two hemodialysis centers were compared with respect to the influence of iron administration on serum ferritin levels. One contributed 35 patients. None of them had received iron therapy except in the form of blood transfusions.

Iron had been administered in function of serum iron levels to the 20 patients from center two. Patients with serum iron concentrations below 60 µg/dl had received iron intravenously. The serum ferritin levels were determined by means of radio-immuno assay (Gamma Dab® ^{125}I-Ferritin kit, Clinical Assays), using crystalline human liver ferritin [23].

Finally, the FEP level was measured in two groups of chronic hemodialysis patients in order to define additional parameters of iron needs in dialysis patients. The first group consisted of 27 patients, who had not received iron therapy except in the form of blood transfusions. The second group consisted of 25 patients, who had received intravenous iron therapy. For the measurement of the FEP to heme ratio, the method described by *Labbe* et al. [24] was used with slight modifications: instead of extracting one drop of whole blood, we extracted 50 µl of packed red blood cells obtained by centrifugating whole blood and sucking off the plasma and the upper layer of red blood cells. The extracted mixture was allowed to stand overnight in the dark at room temperature. In our laboratory [25], the mean FEP to heme ratio was 11 ± 4 (SD) in healthy volunteers. FEP to heme ratios were considered to be pathologically increased when they were 40 or more.

The Wilcoxon signed rank test was used to determine statistical significance and the relationships were evaluated with Spearman rank correlation coefficients (r_s).

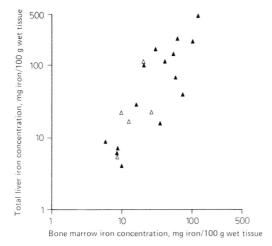

Fig. 3. Liver and bone marrow iron concentrations (AAS). Wet tissue specimens were obtained in deceased patients with severe renal failure (r_s = 0.84, p < 0.001). ▲ = Patients treated with chronic hemodialysis (n = 15); △ = patients without dialysis therapy (n = 5).

Results

The distribution of our severe renal failure patients with respect to cytological bone marrow iron stores is shown in figure 2. These patients had received 2,000 ± 2,700 ml blood (mean ± SD), during the year preceding the bone marrow examinations, but none of them had received iron supplements. Nevertheless, iron stores generally were not depleted (fig. 2). A comparison of bone marrow and liver iron concentrations, determined by means of AAS, showed a good correlation (fig. 3). This, however, did not exclude that in most patients the liver iron levels were higher than the bone marrow iron concentrations, but the reverse situation was observed in others. When comparing Kupffer cell and hepatocyte iron, the disproportionate storage in the different iron compartments was also evident (fig. 4). In some patients hepatocyte iron predominated; while in others Kupffer cell iron was clearly preponderant.

The LAMMA studies, which were performed in 3 patients with clinically, histochemically and chemically established dialysis osteomalacia indicated that iron was present concurrently with aluminum at the osteoid/calcified-bone interface in the first two patients (fig. 5). In the third patient, only aluminum was detected at the osteoid/calcified-bone boundary.

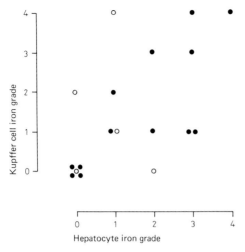

Fig. 4. Comparison between histologically graded liver parenchymal iron content and Kupffer cell iron content in deceased patients with severe renal failure ($r_s = 0.11$, $p < 0.05$). ● = Patients treated with chronic hemodialysis (n = 13); ○ = patients without dialysis therapy (n = 5).

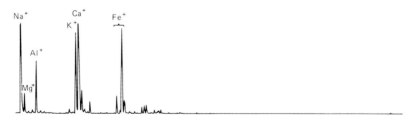

Fig. 5. LAMMA of a bone biopsy from a patient with iron and aluminum overload and dialysis osteomalacia. The mass spectrum corresponds to a region at the osteoid/calcified-bone interface. Important iron and aluminum signals are seen.

In the first patient, the LAMMA technique was also used to define the ultrastructural localization of iron and aluminum in the liver. Iron and aluminum were only detected in electron-dense bodies of hepatocytes (fig. 6) and of Kupffer cells. These electron-dense bodies were identified as lysosomes by means of a histochemical staining method for acid phosphatases [26].

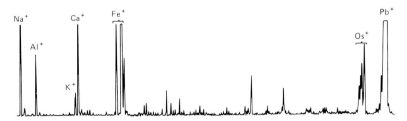

Fig. 6. LAMMA of a liver biopsy from a patient with iron and aluminum overload and dialysis osteomalacia. The mass spectrum, showing large iron and aluminum signals, corresponds to a lysosomal region of a hepatocyte. Osmium and lead signals are due to the fixation and staining procedures, respectively.

Several authors have studied the relationship between serum ferritin levels and iron stores in chronic hemodialysis patients (table II). In view of the relatively close correlation between serum ferritin levels and gradings of reticuloendothelial bone marrow iron, serum ferritin has been proposed as a guide to iron therapy in chronic hemodialysis patients. However, to fulfil this requirement, serum ferritin levels should adequately detect low bone marrow iron stores. Table II indicates that the number of patients presenting low bone marrow iron stores was variable (depending on the criterion of the author) and that serum ferritin levels of these patients were within normal limits in a considerable number of cases. Thus, abnormally low serum ferritin levels are rarely seen in chronic hemodialysis patients. When present, however, they indicate low reticulo endothelial bone marrow iron [27].

Iron administration definitely influences serum ferritin levels. Serum ferritin levels were 333 ± 320 ng/ml (mean ± SD) in a group of chronic hemodialysis patients, who had never received iron therapy, except in the form of blood transfusions (fig. 7). However, patients of another hemodialysis center, who received intravenous iron therapy, showed much higher serum ferritin concentrations of 1,373 ± 767 ng/ml.

In order to determine the beneficial effect of iron therapy upon heme synthesis in chronic hemodialysis patients, FEP to heme ratios were measured. From 27 patients, not receiving iron supplements (except blood transfusions), 2 showed clearly increased FEP to heme ratios. From 25 patients, receiving intravenous iron therapy, 1 presented a considerably increased FEP to heme ratio.

Table II. Serum ferritin levels and iron stores in chronic hemodialysis patients

Reference	Number of chronic dialysis patients studied	Parameters of body iron	Grading scale of bone marrow iron stores	Number of patients with low bone marrow iron grade (criterion of low bone marrow iron grade)		Range of SF levels of patients with low bone marrow iron grade (lower normal limit of the serum ferritin assay used)[1]		Correlation coefficient between bone marrow iron stores and serum ferritin levels
Hussein et al., 1975[5]	44	cBMIS[2]	0–3	4	(0)	10–127	(M 110, F 15)	NM
Beallo et al., 1976[6]	12	cBMIS	0–3	4	(0)	14–35	(12)	NM
Mirahmadi et al., 1977[11]	14	cBMIS	0–7	9	(0–3)	5–100	(NM)	r = 0.771
Aljama et al., 1978[7]	20	hBMIS[3]	0–5	6	(0–0.5)	16–340	(M 32, F 17)	NM
Craswell et al., 1978[9]	28	cBMIS	0–3	3	(0)	13–33	(M 20, F 10)	NM
Bell et al., 1980[14]	55	cBMIS	0–3	42	(0 or 1)	4–127	(<18)	0.884
Milman et al., 1980[16]	31	cBMIS	0–3	19	(0)	6–136	(M 19, F 5)	NM
Birgegård et al., 1981[18]	19	cBMIS	0–3	5	(0)	30–90 U/l	(40 U/l)	NM
Van de Vyver et al., 1982[27]	61	cBMIS-LIS[4]	0–6	15	(0–1)	5–347	(M 20, F 10)	r = 0.78[5]
Ali et al., 1982[2]	36	hBMIS-LIS[6] SIS	[6]0–4	4	(0)	NM–3,994	(M 34, F 17)	r = 0.42

NM = Not mentioned; M = male; F = female.
[1] Expressed in ng/ml, unless otherwise specified.
[2] Cytologically graded bone marrow iron stores.
[3] Histologically graded bone marrow iron stores.
[4] Liver iron stores.
[5] Spearman rank correlation coefficient.
[6] Spleen iron stores.

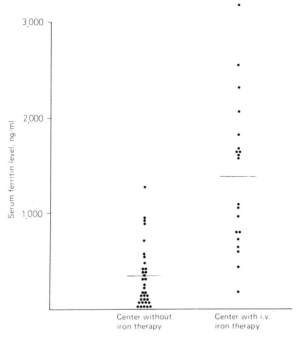

Fig. 7. Serum ferritin levels in chronic hemodialysis patients from 2 centers. Left column = Patients without iron therapy; right column = patients with intravenous iron therapy, according to serum iron levels. Mean serum ferritin level of each group is indicated by a horizontal bar.

Discussion

The study of the patterns of iron storage in severe renal failure is a prerequisite in the evaluation of iron handling in chronic hemodialysis patients. In this study, iron storage was determined at the tissue level with AAS, at the cellular level with histochemical iron staining and at the ultrastructural level with LAMMA.

In most of our patients with severe renal failure, reticulo endothelial bone marrow iron stores were not depleted (fig. 2). Like *Ali* et al. [2], we also noted, however, a disproportionate iron storage in the bone marrow and in the liver in patients with severe renal failure. In fact, while the liver and the bone marrow iron concentrations (AAS of wet tissue specimens) were well correlated, individual patients showed a preferential iron storage either in the liver or in the bone marrow (fig. 3). Moreover, the distribution of iron between the two types of iron storing liver cells (hepatocytes and Kupffer cells) was also variable (fig. 4).

The ultrastructural localization of iron and its spatial relation with other elements was investigated by means of LAMMA. With this technique, iron and aluminum were demonstrated concomitantly in hepatocyte lysosomes, in Kupffer cell lysosomes and at the osteoid/calcified-bone interface in a patient with pronounced iron and aluminum accumulation. These observations confirm and extend the results of other authors, who used other microanalytical procedures [28, 29]. Other examples exist of a similar behavior of iron and aluminum: binding to organic substances, such as deferrioxamine [30] and transferrin [31]; interaction with ferroxidase [32].

The use of serum ferritin levels as a guide for iron therapy in chronic hemodialysis patients is based upon two major suppositions.

Firstly, the amount of stored iron is a good parameter of iron needs. This statement is doubtful, since most normal individuals show minor reticuloendothelial iron in their bone marrow [33].

Second, the close relationship between serum ferritin levels and iron stores, observed in healthy individuals [34], is also existing in severe renal failure. This relationship has been studied using cytologically graded reticuloendothelial bone marrow iron as a parameter of total body iron stores [5, 6, 9, 11, 14, 16, 18].

The relationship, however, between serum ferritin levels and total body iron stores is difficult to determine, in view of the disproportionate iron storage in the two main iron storing organs, the liver and the bone marrow [2, 27]. Consequently, the use of cytologically [5, 6, 9, 11, 14, 16, 18] or histologically [7] graded reticulo endothelial bone marrow iron as a parameter of total body iron stores is questionable.

Although several studies point out that there is a statistically significant correlation between serum ferritin levels and reticuloendothelial bone marow [5–7, 9, 11, 14, 16, 18, 27], and between serum ferritin levels and liver iron [2, 27], serum ferritin levels do not seem appropriate to uncover patients with depleted bone marrow iron stores. Undoubtedly, these are the patients, who might require iron therapy. In fact, abnormally low serum ferritin levels are associated with absent reticuloendothelial bone marrow iron. However, the reverse is not true; most patients without visible iron in their bone marrow macrophages show normal serum ferritin levels. Increasing the diagnostic threshold of serum ferritin levels for chronic hemodialysis patients, as proposed by some authors, cannot overcome this problem.

It should be noted that some of these authors do not mention the serum ferritin kit used. This is important, however, since the results of serum ferritin measurements depend largely upon the radioimmunoassay kit used [35]. Furthermore, many commercial methods do not lend themselves to detect abnormally low serum ferritin levels, since standards with serum ferritin concentrations below the lower normal limit are not provided [36].

Serum ferritin levels of chronic hemodialysis patients without iron therapy (except blood transfusions) were normal to high, while those of patients receiving intravenous iron therapy were markedly elevated in most cases (fig. 7). Considerable amounts of bone marrow storage iron were present in most of our patients (fig. 2). Accepting that a good statistical relationship exists between serum ferritin levels and the amount of bone marrow storage iron [27], we may anticipate that the elevated serum ferritin levels reflect greatly increased iron stores after intravenous iron.

In chronic hemodialysis patients not receiving iron therapy, abnormally elevated FEP to heme ratios were rarely observed. This is in accordance with observations of other authors in patients with severe renal failure [37,38]. This might indicate the absence of clinically important iron deficiency [39].

From these results some conclusions, concerning patients with severe renal failure, may be inferred: (1) Iron is disproportionately stored in the different bone marrow and liver storage compartments. (2) In some patients, showing both iron and aluminum accumulation , the two elements are detected concurrently with LAMMA in hepatocyte lysosomes, Kupffer cell lysosomes and at the osteoid/calcified-bone interface. (3) Abnormally low serum ferritin levels correspond to abnormally low bone marrow iron stores. From higher serum ferritin levels, however, no unequivocal conclusions can be drawn.

Finally, in our opinion, iron supply to chronic hemodialysis patients, especially to those being transfused, can be questioned based on the following arguments: (1) Features of iron deficiency anemia, such as hypochromic microcytic anemia [40], or increased FEP to heme ratios [39], are rarely seen in severe renal failure. (2) Chronic dialysis patients receive blood transfusions (containing considerable amounts of iron) to treat anemias, which are not related to iron deficiency or in the context of a pretransplant program. (3) Iron stores generally are not depleted in chronic hemodialysis patients not receiving iron therapy (except blood transfusions). (4) The feedback mechanism, consisting of increased gastrointestinal iron absorption in patients with iron deficiency, has been demonstrated in chronic hemodialysis patients [41]. (5) The undesirable effects of excessive iron storage have been documented in patients with chronic hemodialysis [3, 4]. Nevertheless, iron depletion should be anticipated in chronic hemodialysis patients, who are not transfused and who present a serum ferritin level below the lower normal limit of the assay kit used. Whenever iron supplements need to be administered to dialysis patients, the oral route should be chosen.

Acknowledgement

We are most grateful to all collaborating nephrologists: Dr. *I. Becaus*, Dr. *V. Bosteels*, Dr. *J. Boelaert*, Dr. *R. Hombrouckx*, Dr. *H. Janssen*, Dr. *R. Lins*, Dr. *M. Segaert*, Dr. *G. Verpooten*, and Dr. *D. Walb*. In addition, we wish to express our thanks to Mrs. *A. Grootveld* for secreterial help.

References

1   Edwards, M.S.; Pegrum, G.D.; Curtis, J.R.: Iron therapy in patients on maintenance haemodialysis. Lancet *ii*: 491−493 (1970).
2   Ali, M.; Rigolosi, R.; Fayemi, A.O.; Braun, E.V.; Frascino, F.; Singer, R.: Failure of serum ferritin levels to predict bonemarrow iron content after intravenous iron-dextran therapy. Lancet *i*: 652−655 (1982).
3   Kothari, T.; Swamy, A.P.; Lee, J.C.K.; Mangla, J.C.; Cestero R.V.M.: Hepatic hemosiderosis in maintenance hemodialysis (MHD) patients. Dig. Dis. Sci. *25*: 363−368 (1980).
4   Bregman, H.; Gelfand, M.C.; Winchester, J.F.; Manz, H.J.; Knepshield, J.H.; Schreiner, G.E.: Iron-overload-associated myopathy in patients on maintenance haemodialysis. A histocompatibility-linked disorder. Lancet *ii*: 882−885 (1980).
5   Hussein, S.; Prieto, J.; O'Shea, M.; Hoffbrand, A.V.; Baillod, R.A.; Moorhead, J.F.: Serum ferritin assay and iron status in chronic renal failure and haemodialysis. Br. med. J. *i*: 546−548 (1975).
6   Beallo, R.; Dallman, P.R.; Schoenfeld, P.Y.; Humphreys, M.H.: Serum ferritin and iron deficiency in patients on chronic hemodialysis. Trans. Am. Soc. artif. internal Organs *22*: 73−79 (1976).
7   Aljama, P.; Ward, M.K.; Pierides, A.M.; Eastham, E.J.; Ellis, H.A.; Feest, T.G.; Conceicao, S.; Kerr, D.N.S.: Serum ferritin concentration: a reliable guide to iron overload in uremic and hemodialyzed patients. Clin. Nephrol. *10*: 101−104 (1978).

8 Eschbach, J.W.; Cook, J.D.; Scribner, B.H.; Finch, C.A.: Iron balance in hemodialysis patients. Ann. intern. Med. *87*: 710–713 (1977).

9 Craswell, P.; Hunt, F.; Davies, L.; Russo, A.; Goethart, J.; Halliday, J.: Serum ferritin as an index of body iron stores in patients on chronic haemodialysis. Aust. N.Z.J. Med. *8*: 38–42 (1978).

10 Eschbach, J.W.; Cook, J.D.: Quantitating iron balance in hemodialysis patients. Trans. Am. Soc. artif. internal Organs *23*: 54–58 (1977).

11 Mirahmadi, K.S.; Paul, W.L.; Winer, R.L.; Nosratolah, D.V.; Byer, B.; Gorman, J.T.; Rosen, S.M.: Serum ferritin level. Determinant of iron requirement in hemodialysis patients. J. Am. med. Ass. *238*: 601–603 (1977).

12 Ellis, D.: Serum ferritin compared with other indices of iron status in children and teenagers undergoing maintenance hemodialysis. Clin. Chem. *25*: 741–744 (1979).

13 Parker, P.A.; Izard, M.W.; Maher, J.F.: Therapy of iron deficiency anemia in patients on maintenance dialysis. Nephron *23*: 181–186 (1979).

14 Bell, J.D.; Kincaid, W.R.; Morgan, R.G.; Bunce, H.; Alperin, J.B.; Sarles, H.E.; Remmers, A.R.: Serum ferritin assay and bonemarrow iron stores in patients on maintenance hemodialysis. Kidney int. *17*: 237–241 (1980).

15 Lynn, K.L.; Mitchell, T.R.; Schepperd, J.: Serum ferritin concentration in patients receiving maintenance hemodialysis. Clin. Nephrol. *14*: 124–127 (1980).

16 Milman, N.; Christensen, T.E.; Pedersen, N.S.; Visfeldt, J.: Serum ferritin and bone marrow iron in non-dialysis, peritoneal dialysis and hemodialysis patients with chronic renal failure. Acta med. scand. *207*: 201–205 (1980).

17 Müller, H.A.G.; Schneider, H.; Hövelborn, U.; Streicher, E.: Ferritin: a reliable indicator of iron supplementation in patients on chronic hemodialysis/hemofiltration treatment? Artif. Organs *5*: 168–174 (1981).

18 Birgegård, G.; Nilsson, P.; Wide, L.: Regulation of iron therapy by S-ferritin estimations in patients on chronic hemodialysis. Scand. J. Urol. Nephrol. *15*: 69–72 (1981).

19 Meunier, P.; Courpron, P.; Edouard, C.; Bernard, J.; Bringuier; Vignon, G.: Physiological senile involution and pathological rarefaction of bone. Quantitative and comparative histological data. Clin. Endocr. Metab. *2*: 239–256 (1973).

20 Gale, E.; Torrance, J.; Bothwell, T.: The quantitative estimation of total iron stores in human bone marrow. J. clin. Invest. *42*: 1076–1082 (1963).

21 Scheuer, P.J.; Williams, R.; Muir, A.R.: Hepatic pathology in relatives of patients with hemochromatosis. J. Path. Bact. *84*: 53–64 (1962).

22 Schmidt, P.F.; Fromme, H.G.; Pfefferkorn, G.: LAMMA-investigations of biological and medical specimens. Scanning Electron Microsc. *II*: 623–634 (1980).

23 Hazard, J.T.; Yokota, M.; Arosio, P.; Drysdale, J.W.: Immunologic differences in human isoferritins. Implications for immunologic quantitation of serum ferritin. Blood 49: 139-146 (1977).

24 Labbe, R.F.; Finch, C.A.; Smith, N.J.; Doan, R.N.; Sood, S.K.; Madan, N.: Erythrocyte protoporphyrin/heme ratio in the assessment of iron status. Clin. Chem. *25*: 87–92 (1979).

25 Jackson, K.W.: Interlaboratory comparison of results of erythrocyte protoporphyrin analysis. Clin. Chem. *24*: 2135–2138 (1979).

26 De Jong, A.S.H.; Hak, T.J.; Van Duyn, P.; Daems, W.T.: A new dynamic model system for the study of capture reactions for diffusible compounds in cytochemistry. II.

Effect of the composition of the incubation medium on the trapping of phosphate ions in acid phosphatase cytochemistry. Histochem. J. *11*: 145−161 (1979).

27   Van de Vyver, F.L.; Vanheule, A.O.; Majelyne, W.M.; D'Haese, P.; Blockx, P.P.; Bekaert, A.B.; Buyssens, N.; De Keersmaecker, W.; De Broe, M.E.: Serum ferritin as a guide for iron stores in patients with severe renal failure. Kidney int (submitted).

28   Galle, P.; Giudicelli, C.P.: Toxicité de l'aluminium pour l'hépatocyte. Localisation ultrastructurale et micro-analyse des dépôts. Nouv. Presse méd. *11*: 1123−1125 (1982).

29   Brown, D.J.; Dawborn, J.K.; Ham, K.N.; Xipell, J.M.: Treatment of dialysis osteomalacia with desferrioxamine. Lancet *ii*: 343−345 (1982).

30   Ackrill, P.; Ralston, A.J.; Day, J.P.; Hodge, K.C.: Successful removal of aluminium from a patient with dialysis encephalopathy. Lancet *ii*: 692−693 (1980).

31   Donovan, J.W.; Ross, K.D.: Nonequivalence of the metal binding sites of conalbumin. Calorimetric and Spectrophotometric studies of aluminium binding. J. biol. Chem. *250*: 6022−6025 (1975).

32   Huber, C.T.; Frieden, E.: The inhibition of ferroxidase by trivalent and other metal ions. J. biol. Chem. *245*: 3979−3984 (1970).

33   Lundin, P.; Persson, E.; Weinfeld, A.: Comparison of hemosiderin estimation in bone marrow sections and bone marrow smears. Acta med. scand. *175*: 383−390 (1964).

34   Jacobs, A.; Miller, F.; Worwood, M.; Beamish, M.R.; Wardrop, C.A.: Ferritin in the serum of normal subjects and patients with iron deficiency and iron overload. Br. med. J. *iv*: 206−208 (1972).

35   Werner, E.; Kaltwasser, J.P.: Nachweisverfahren zur Serumferritinbestimmung, pp. 34−55 (Springer, Berlin 1980).

36   Ng, R.H.; Statland, B.E.: Lack of ferritin concentration at the decision level among commercial quality-control materials. Clin. Chem. *29*: 580 (1983).

37   Vlassopoulos, K.; Melissinos, K.; Drivas, G.: The erythrocyte protoporphyrin in chronic renal failure. Clinica chim. Acta *65*: 389−392 (1975).

38   Linkesch, W.; Stummvoll, H.K.; Wolf, A.; Müller, M.: Heme synthesis in anemia of the uremic state. Israel J. med. Scis *14*: 1173−1176 (1978).

39   Piomelli, S.; Brickman, A.; Carlos, E.: Rapid diagnosis of iron deficiency by measurement of free erythrocyte porphyrins and hemoglobin: the FEP/hemoglobin ratio. Pediatrics, Springfield *57*: 136−141 (1976).

40   Bainton, D.F.; Finch, C.A.: The diagnosis of iron deficiency anemia. Am. J. Med. *37*: 62−70 (1964).

41   Eschbach, J.W.; Cook, J.D.; Scribner, B.H.; Finch, C.A.: Iron balance in hemodialysis patients. Ann. intern. Med. *87*: 710−713 (1977).

F. Van de Vyver, MD, p/a Prof. Dr. M.E. De Broe, Dept. of Nephrology-Hypertension, University Hospital Antwerp, Wilrijkstraat 10, B-2520 Edegem (Belgium)

Contr. Nephrol., vol. 38, pp. 167–173 (Karger, Basel 1984)

Therapy and Monitoring of Hypersiderosis in Chronic Renal Insufficiency

M. Hilfenhaus[a], K.-M. Koch[a], P.B. Bechstein[b], H. Schmidt[b], W. Fassbinder[b], C.A. Baldamus[b]

[a]Department of Nephrology, University of Hannover Medical School, Hannover, FRG;
[b]Department of Nephrology, University Clinic Frankfurt am Main, FRG

Causes of Hemosiderosis

In patients with preterminal renal failure without blood transfusions and iron substitution hemosiderosis is absent [7]. Because of occult intestinal blood loss and reduced iron intake due to protein restriction iron stores may even be diminished [8]. The exception is the rare patient who, because of severe renal anemia, is in need of frequent blood transfusions already in the preterminal stage of renal disease. In contrast, in patients on regular hemodialysis hemosiderosis is a more common finding:

(1) With progression of renal disease to the terminal stage, in a small percentage of patients anemia may worsen to such an extent that regular blood transfusions are required. This is especially the case in bilaterally nephrectomized patients. Furthermore due to a reduced tolerance to even a moderate degree of anemia older hemodialysis patients with severe arteriosclerosis may be in need of regular transfusions. Only in these groups of end-stage renal disease patients with transfusional iron overload, development of hemosiderosis is an inevitable event.

(2) A further cause for hemosiderosis in regular hemodialysis patients is excessive substitution of dialysis-related iron losses. This applies especially to parenteral iron application. However, in susceptible patients even orally administrated iron has been reported to result in hemosiderosis [3]. In contrast to transfusional iron overload, hemosiderosis due to iron substitution is preventable by monitoring of body iron stores.

Consequences of Hemosiderosis

Excessive transfusional iron overload in patients with thalassemia and other forms of nonrenal chronic anemia is accompanied by severe hemosiderosis with organ damage. Heart failure due to myocardial iron deposition is the most common cause of death in thalassemia [10]. Cirrhosis of the liver and endocrinopathies are further consequences of hemosiderosis in these patients [13].

In regular hemodialysis patients pathological iron deposition has been demonstrated in bone marrow, liver (reticuloendothelial and parenchymal deposits), spleen, myocardium and skeletal muscle [1, 3, 7]. However, so far only myopathy [3] and histological abnormalities of the liver [7] — in our experience accompanied by elevated transaminases — have been described as clinical consequences of hemosiderosis in regular hemodialysis patients. In case of myopathy a predisposing factor was the existence of one or more of the hemochromatosis alleles HLA A_3, B_7 and B_{14} [3].

In polytransfused patients without renal disease clinically overt cardiomyopathy and endocrinopathy have been limited to patients with total iron loads above 60 g, which is equivalent to approximately one transfusion per week for 5—6 years [10]. This explains why these complications of hemosiderosis have not yet been seen in regular hemodialysis where patients are rarely in need of frequent transfusions for such long periods of time.

Monitoring of Body Iron Stores

Several investigators [2, 4, 7] were able to demonstrate that serum ferritin determination — as in patients without renal disease — is the most reliable and easily accessible method to quantify body iron stores in regular hemodialysis patients. The correlation between magnitude of body iron stores and serum ferritin concentration may be disturbed in patients with liver disease or inflammation [9], as these patients have inappropriately high serum ferritin levels. For instance, patients with liver disease and absent bone marrow iron may have normal serum ferritin levels. Another limitation of serum ferritin as a measure of iron stores is that it does not distinguish between parenchymal and reticuloendothelial iron. In patients without renal disease and elevated serum ferritin levels, determination of transferrin saturation helps to locate iron stores, as a transferrin saturation above 70% indicates parenchymal loading [6]. So far it is unknown whether this relation also holds for patients with renal disease.

Therapy

In case of uncomplicated hemosiderosis due to inadequate iron supplementation, normalization of iron stores is most easily achieved in regular hemodialysis patients by discontinuation of iron substitution. Dialysis-related blood loss will gradually reduce iron stores towards normal, recognizable by decreasing serum ferritin levels. Only when excessive hemosiderosis is accompanied by clinical or biochemical signs of organ damage − for instance elevated transaminases not attributable to other toxic or inflammatory liver disturbances − more rigorous measures are indicated. Phlebotomy is limited to those hemodialysis patients who have sufficient erythropoiesis with hematocrits above 30% or to patients with significant improvement of anemia following transplantation.

The following case history describes the effectiveness of discontinuation of iron therapy during regular dialysis treatment as well as of phlebotomy following transplantation in the same patient:

R.W., male, 31 years. HLA A_2, A_3, B_{12}, BW 18. Terminal renal failure due to chronic glomerulonephritis. 1970−1980: Regular dialysis treatment (RDT). 1970−1978: 16 g Fe i.v., 1 g Fe orally. 1978: Serum ferritin 4,800 μg/l, Hct 30%, SGOT and SGPT constantly elevated, maximal values 160 and 180 U/l, respectively. AUSH-Ag negative, no CMV titer. Liver biopsy: severe parenchymal and reticuloendothelial siderosis. 1978: Discontinuation of iron substitution. 1980: Serum ferritin 1,580 μg/l, maximum SGOT 50 U/l, SGPT normal. 1980: Successful cadaveric transplantation. March 1981 till February 1983: 28 phlebotomies with a total volume of 14 liters. February 1983: Serum ferritin 380 μg/l, Hct 35.6%. SGOT and SGPT constantly normal.

In RDT patients with severe hemosiderosis due to frequent transfusions who cannot be transplanted, desferrioxamine (DFO) treatment has to be considered. Iron chelated by DFO in patients without renal disease is excreted as ferrioxamine in urine and to a lesser degree in feces [14]. While unchelated iron is rejected, ferrioxamine passes the dialysis membrane [12]. In vitro studies showed ferrioxamine dialysances to be higher with acrylonitrile-Co-polymer membranes than with cellulose membranes [12]. In vivo studies in hemodialysis patients demonstrated that dependent upon DFO dosis (0.5−4 g parenteral/dialysis), iron removed in dialysate varies between 5.8 and 109 mg/dialysis treatment [7, 12].

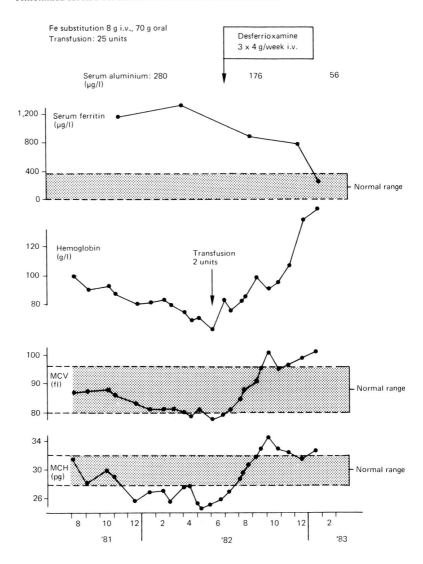

Fig. 1. The effect of long-term DFO treatment on serum ferritin, serum aluminum and anemia in a patient (W.K., male, 48 years) on regular hemodialysis for 6 years with aluminum-related osteomalacia and iron overload. MCV = Mean corpuscular volume; MCH = mean corpuscular hemoglobin.

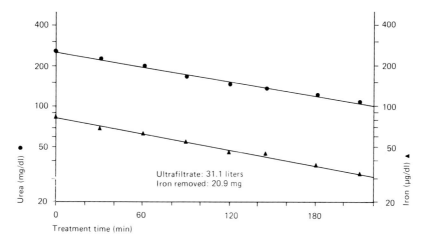

Fig. 2. Ultrafiltrate urea and iron concentration during hemofiltration following 1 g DFO i.v. Patient M.H., female, 44 kg body weight, serum ferritin 8,300 μg/l.

The long-term effect of DFO treatment in an RDT patient with iron overload is shown in figure 1. This patient was treated with DFO because of aluminum-related osteomalacia. 4 g of DFO were infused during the last hour of every hemodialysis for 6 months. His serum ferritin level dropped from 1,316 μg/l before treatment to 239 μg/l after treatment. At the same time serum aluminum levels decreased and aluminum-related microcytotic hypochromic anemia improved dramatically.

In hemofiltration DFO-chelated iron is also removed effectively (fig. 2). In an end-stage renal disease patient with a heavy iron overload due to multiple transfusions we infused 1 g of DFO over 45 min 1 h before hemofiltration treatment. In 31.3 liters of ultrafiltrate a total of 20.9 mg of iron was removed. Provided sieving coefficients are equal, the parallel decrease of urea and Fe concentration in the ultrafiltrate indicates that the volume of distribution of DFO is similar to that of urea, i.e. total body water. In hemosiderotic patients on peritoneal dialysis iron can also be removed effectively by applying DFO parenterally or intraperitoneally. In a CAPD patient either 3 × 1.5 g DFO i.v./week or 250 mg DFO/l of dialysate removed 78 and 88 mg iron/week, respectively [5]. In addition to enabling iron removal by dialytic procedures DFO can also cause an up to twofold increase in fecal iron excretion in end-stage renal disease patients [7].

Several investigators [10, 11, 14] were able to demonstrate that in regard to iron removal continuous infusion of DFO is superior to applying equal doses of DFO over shorter periods of time. This is explained by the existence of a rapidly renewed labile iron pool susceptible to chelation. Constant infusion in contrast to bolus injection would cause continuous exposure of the chelator to iron molecules passing through the pool [10]. Whether from these observations in patients without renal disease it can be concluded that continuous i.v. infusion of DFO during dialysis is superior to bolus injection is still uncertain, as there exist no quantified data collected in RDT patients regarding this issue.

Reported acute side effects of DFO include allergic reactions, bradycardia and tachycardia, hyper- and hypotension, headache and rigors. A recognized but rare complication of long-term application is reversible cataract [10]. Because of these side effects DFO treatment should only be considered in end-stage renal disease patients when other measures of treatment of iron overload are ineffective.

Summary and Conclusions

(1) In RDT hemosiderosis appears to be an inevitable complication only in the small number of patients in need of frequent transfusions.

(2) To prevent clinical consequences (e.g. cardiomyopathy) known from polytransfused patients without renal disease, transplantation should be considered in RDT patients in need of frequent transfusions.

(3) Iron substitution − preferably oral − to replace dialysis-related iron loss does not cause clinically significant hemosiderosis provided iron stores are monitored adequately.

(4) A sufficient method of controlling iron stores in RDT patients under iron substitution or regular transfusion therapy is a twice annual determination of serum ferritin concentration.

(5) The treatment of choice for hemosiderosis in nontransfused RDT patients is discontinuation of iron substitution.

(6) When polytransfused RDT patients with severe hemosiderosis cannot be transplanted and submitted consecutively to phlebotomy, DFO treatment is indicated.

(7) Quantitative data regarding optimal dosage and application of DFO in RDT patients are not yet available. Constant infusion of DFO during hemodialysis may be superior to bolus application.

References

1 Ali, M.; Rigolosi, R.; Fayemi, A.Ö.; Braun, E.V.; Frascino, J.; Singer, R.: Failure of serum ferritin levels to predict bone-marrow iron content after intravenous iron-dextran therapy. Lancet *i*: 652–655 (1982).

2 Bechstein, R.-B.; Kaltwasser, J.B.; Koch, K.-M.; Werner, E.: Die Bedeutung der Serumferritinbestimmung zur Ermittlung der Eisenspeicher in der chronischen Niereninsuffizienz; in Kaltwasser, Werner, Serumferritin, p. 259 (Springer, Berlin 1980).

3 Bregman, H.; Gelfand, M.C.; Winchester, J.F.; Manz, H.J.; Knepshield, J.H.; Schreiner, G.E.: Iron-overload-associated myopathy in patients on maintenance haemodialysis: a histo-compatibility-linked disorder. Lancet *ii*: 882–885 (1980).

4 Eschbach, J.W.; Cook, J.D.; Scribner, B.H.; Finch, C.A.: Iron balance in hemodialysis patients. Ann. intern. Med. *87*: 710–713 (1977).

5 Falk, R.J.; Mattern, W.D.; Lamanna, R.W.; Parker, N.C.; Cross, R.E.: Iron removal during CAPD (Abstract). Am. Soc. Nephrol., 14th Annu. Meet., 1981, p. 39A.

6 Finch, C.A.: The detection of iron overload. New Engl. J. Med. *307*: 1702–1703 (1982).

7 Gokal, R.; Millard, P.R.; Weatherall, D.J.; Callender, S.T.E.; Ledingham, J.G.G.; Oliver, D.O.: Iron metabolism in haemodialysis patients. Q. Jl. Med. *68*: 369–391 (1979).

8 Koch, K.-M.; Bechstein, P.B.; Fassbinder, W.; Kaltwasser, P.; Schoeppe, W.; Werner, E.: Occult blood loss and iron balance in chronic renal failure. EDTA Proc. *12*: 362–369 (1975).

9 Lipschitz, D.A.; Cook, J.D.; Finch, C.A.: A clinical evaluation of serum ferritin as an index of iron stores. New Engl. J. Med. *290*: 1213–1216 (1974).

10 Modell, B.: Advances in the use of iron-chelating agents for the treatment of iron over-load. Prog. Hemat. *11*: 267–312 (1979).

11 Propper, R.D.; Shurin, S.B.; Nathan, D.G.: Reassessment of the use of desfer-rioxamine B in iron overload. New Engl. J. Med. *294*: 1421–1423 (1976).

12 Rembold, C.M.; Krumlovsky, F.A.; Roxe, D.M.; Fitzsimmons, E.; Greco, F. del: Treatment of hemodialysis hemosiderosis with desferrioxamine. Trans. Am. Soc. artif, internal Organs *28*: 621–626 (1982).

13 Schafer, A.I.; Cheron, R.B.; Dluhy, R.; Cooper, B.; Gleason, R.E.; Soeldner, J.S.; Bunn, H.F.: Clinical consequences of acquired transfusional iron overload in adults. New Engl. J. Med. *304*: 319–324 (1981).

14 Weatherall, D.J.; Pippard, M.J.; Callender, S.T.: Iron loading in thalassemia. Five years with the pump. New Engl. J. Med. *308*: 456–457 (1983).

M. Hilfenhaus, MD, Abteilung Nephrologie, Medizinische Hochschule Hannover, D-3000 Hannover (FRG)

Contr. Nephrol., vol. 38, p. 174 (Karger, Basel 1984)

Discussion: Iron Metabolism

By means of ferrokinetic data it can be concluded that progressive loss of renal function results in an erythropoetin-deficient hypoproliferative anemia and increasing iron stores. Iron overload, e.g. by transfusions, is capable of further suppression of the erythropoesis. The different levels of hemoglobin seen in ESRD patients with similar degrees of uremia seem to correlate with different levels of erythropoetin production, inhibitors of erythropoesis may modulate this correlation, but this is speculative. Substitution of iron losses can be accomplished via the oral route, as iron absorption is normal in individuals on dialysis. On the other hand, it might be impossible to give them enough iron to compensate for greater losses, so parenteral iron application is equally feasible without influence on its utilisation. Measurements of serum ferritin concentrations reliably reflect iron stores in ESRD patients with a high correlation even to liver iron concentrations. DFO application for treatment of iron overload hepatopathy remains controversial on the basis of a CAT scan liver densitometry for estimation of liver iron stores. On the other hand, potential hazards of remittent DFO application are unclear. DFO treatment with subcutaneous application is followed by a greater iron elimination during HF than after other routes of application (e.g., i.v., i.m.) The indication for starting DFO treatment in ESRD patients in order to avoid irreversible organ damage may be seen if transfused iron surmounts 25 g.

Dr. *E. Streicher, Stuttgart*

Magnesium Metabolism

Contr. Nephrol., vol. 38, pp. 175–184 (Karger, Basel 1984)

Magnesium Homeostasis in Patients with Renal Failure

Shaul G. Massry

Division of Nephrology and Department of Medicine, University of Southern Californias School of Medicine, Los Angeles, Calif., USA

Renal failure may be associated with disturbances in several aspects of magnesium metabolism. These include the renal handling of magnesium, its concentration in blood, tissue content of this ion and its intestinal absorption and balance.

Renal Handling of Magnesium

Patients with advanced renal failure display a significant reduction in their urinary excretion of magnesium [1–4]. We evaluated the 24-hour urinary excretion of magnesium in 50 patients with creatinine clearances ranging between 1 and 30 ml/min; it varied between 12 and 133 mg with a mean of 57 ± 4 (SE) mg [4]. Two-thirds of the patients had hypomagnesiuria while the rest had either normal or increased excretion of magnesium. In uremic patients with salt wasting such as those with chronic pyelonephritis, the 24-hour urinary excretion of magnesium may be normal or high [4] and renal magnesium wasting has been reported in a few such patients [1].

The fraction of filtered magnesium excreted rises as renal insufficiency progresses [3–7], and the increment is more marked when the glomerular filtration rate is less than 10 ml/min (fig. 1, 2). There is a positive and significant correlation between the fraction of filtered magnesium excreted and that of sodium in patients with glomerular filtration below 40 ml/min (fig. 3) [5] and in dogs with experimental renal failure [7]. The mechanisms responsible for the alteration in the renal handling of magnesium in chronic renal failure are not elucidated. They, however, reflect both the extrarenal and intrarenal adaptive processes in response to progressive nephron loss

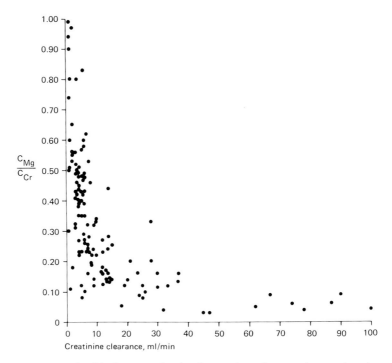

Fig. 1. Relationship between fractional excretion of magnesium and endogenous creatinine clearance in patients with chronic renal disease. Each point represents individual subject [by permission from *Coburn* et al., 6].

with the overall goal being the maintenance of magnesium homeostasis within the normal limits.

We have also evaluated the renal handling of magnesium during the diuretic phase of acute renal failure in 10 patients. The fraction of filtered magnesium excreted is increased and there is a positive and significant correlation between it and that of sodium.

Serum Magnesium in Renal Failure

Acute Renal Failure

We have studied the total and diffusible concentrations of magnesium in the blood of 10 patients with acute renal failure [8] (fig. 4). Hypermag-

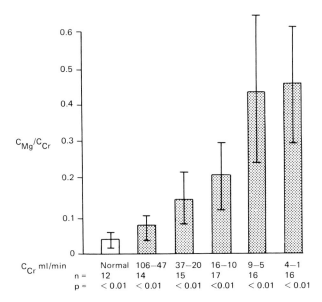

Fig. 2. Mean and SD values for the fractional excretion of filtered magnesium (C_{Mg}/C_{cr}) at different levels of creatinine clearance (C_{cr}). n = Number of patients; p = relation between normal subjects and patients as determined by t test [by permission from *Popovtzer* et al., 5].

nesemia was present in all but 1 patient during the oliguric phase of the illness. The highest values observed in the various patients ranged between 2.2 and 4.6 mg/dl. During the diuretic phase, the levels of magnesium in blood fell to normal or slightly below normal, and they were normal after recovery of renal function. There were no significant changes in the percent diffusibility of blood magnesium, and, therefore, the changes in diffusible magnesium level reflected the alterations in its total concentration.

Chronic Renal Failure

The blood levels of magnesium are usually normal in patients with early renal failure but distinct hypermagnesemia is common in patients with advanced renal failure [6]. It should be mentioned that hypomagnesemia has also been encountered in some patients with chronic renal failure [9–11]. The relationship between the levels of serum magnesium and the degree of renal insufficiency in a large number of patients with creatinine clearance rates below 30 ml/min is depicted in figure 5. Chronic renal failure, as in the case of acute renal failure, did not alter the diffusibility of

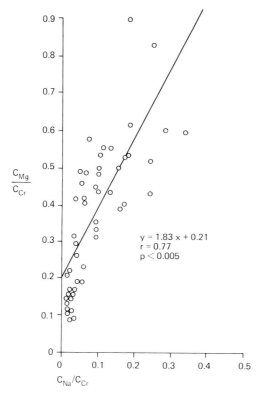

$$y = 1.83 x + 0.21$$
$$r = 0.77$$
$$p < 0.005$$

Fig. 3. The relationship between fractional excretion of magnesium (C_{Mg}/C_{cr}) and that of sodium (C_{Na}/C_{cr}) in patients with renal failure. Each point represents 1 patient [by permission from *Popovtzer* et al., 4].

blood magnesium. Indeed, the percent age of serum magnesium which is not bound to protein was $76 \pm 8\%$, a value which is no different from the $75 \pm 9\%$ observed in normals [6]. Abrupt increments in serum magnesium occur when renal failure patients consume magnesium-containing antacids or laxatives [1].

The levels of serum magnesium in patients undergoing hemodialysis are related to the concentration of magnesium in dialysate as well as to the dietary intake of this ion. Magnesium readily crosses the dialysis membrane, and its movement depends upon the gradient between the concentration of diffusible magnesium in blood and the concentration of magnesium in dialysate [12]. *Schmidt* et al. [13] reported total magnesium losses

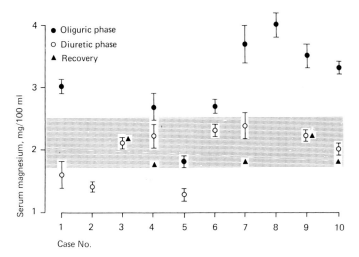

Fig. 4. The levels of serum magnesium in patients with acute renal failure. Each data point represents the mean ± SE of multiple measurements. Closed circles represent values during oliguric phase of acute renal failure; open circles represent data during the diuretic phase and triangles depict values after recovery of renal function. The shaded area shows the normal range. Based on data from *Massry* et al. [8].

as high as 700 mg per dialysis when the dialysate magnesium was 0.27 mg/dl. The importance of dialysate magnesium concentrations in determining the predialysis blood magnesium concentration is demonstrated by our observations in patients treated in two separate dialysis centers with one utilizing dialysate containing 0.6 mg of magnesium/dl and the other 1.9 mg/dl; predialysis blood magnesium level ranged between 1.7 and 2.5 mg/dl and between 3.0 and 5.0 mg/dl in the two centers, respectively [6]. *Blomfield* et al. [14] reported similar observations.

Tissue Content of Magnesium in Chronic Renal Failure

Red Blood Cells (RBC)

The magnesium content of the RBC of the uremic patients treated with maintenance hemodialysis is usually higher than that of normals [13] and RBC magnesium in these patients correlates well with the concentration of magnesium in their blood [14].

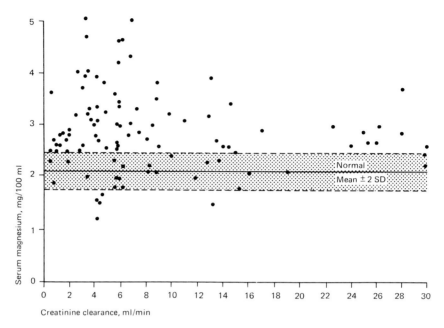

Fig. 5. Relationship between serum magnesium concentration and creatinine clearance rate in patients with chronic renal disease. Each symbol represents single patients [by permission from *Coburn* et al., 6].

Skin

The magnesium content of the skin of dialysis patients is affected by the concentrations of magnesium in dialysate. We have measured the magnesium content in the skin of two populations of patients treated with hemodialysis for periods of 2 months to 5 years with dialysate containing magnesium in concentrations of either 1.8 or 0.6 mg/dl. Although there was an overlap between the individual values, the skin content of magnesium was significantly higher (p < 0.01) in the group treated with dialysate containing 1.8 mg/dl [15].

Muscle

Normal, low or elevated magnesium content in skeletal muscle of patients with chronic renal failure has been reported [16, 17]. *Lim* et al. [16] found that the mean magnesium content in the muscles of nine uremic patients (55.0 ± 7.4 (SE) mEq/kg of dry fat free solids) was significantly lower

($p < 0.05$) than that of normal subjects (71.8 ± 2.5 mEq/kg of dry fat free solids). The magnesium content in the muscles of patients treated with hemodialysis was not different from that observed in the nondialyzed patients. On the other hand, *Contiguglia* et al. [17] reported that the magnesium contents of muscle from normal and uremic patients were no different, 7.5 ± 8.6 and 80.9 ± 14.3 mEq/kg of fat-free solids, respectively.

Bone

The magnesium content of bone in uremic patients is increased. *Contiguglia* et al. [17] found that the magnesium content of both cortical and trabecular bone was increased by 66%. These observations were later confirmed by *Berlyne* et al. [18]. Bone contains two distinct magnesium pools: one is rapidly exchangeable and constitutes 30% of total bone magnesium and the other is nonexchangeable; in patients with uremia, the excess magnesium in bone is distributed in both pools [19]. The hypermagnesemia of renal failure is the most likely cause responsible for the increase in bone magnesium.

Intestinal Absorption of Magnesium in Renal Failure

The usual diet in the United States provides $300-350$ mg of magnesium per day [20–22]. About $25-60\%$ of ingested magnesium is absorbed by the gut. This estimation is derived from measurement of fecal magnesium which ranges between 40 and 70% of the amount ingested [20–23], and from observations that the part of fecal magnesium contributed by endogenous intestinal secretion is very small ($12-24$ mg/day) [24]. In man, most magnesium absorption occurs in the small intestine [25] but magnesium is also absorbed by the large bowel [26].

There is no convincing data for the presence of adaptation in magnesium absorption in relation to habitual dietary intake of this ion or in relation to the body's needs for magnesium. Thus, excess dietary magnesium is readily absorbed, and any surfeit is excreted by the kidney [27]. Conversely, the kidney efficiently conserves magnesium when dietary intake of this mineral is reduced [28, 29]. With impaired renal function, the kidney's capacity to excrete a magnesium load is impaired, making it apparent why marked alterations in magnesium homeostasis may occur in advanced renal failure.

Data in man suggest that high dietary intake of calcium reduces intestinal absorption of magnesium. *Heaton* et al. [30] found that an increase in calcium intake from 1,500 to 3,800 mg/day was associated with a 25% increase in fecal magnesium and 15% decrease in urinary magnesium. *Clarkson* et al. [31] found similar effects of high dietary calcium.

The effect of vitamin D on intestinal absorption of magnesium in man is not well studied. *Heaton* et al. [30] found that fecal magnesium was reduced in 4 of 6 patients treated with either vitamin D_2 or dihydrotachysterol. On the other hand, *Brickman* et al. [32] reported that administration of 1,25-dihydroxyvitamin D_3 in doses of 0.7−2.7 g/day for 10 days to 3 normal subjects, led to a significant decrease in fecal magnesium in only 1 case, despite a substantial effect on calcium absorption in all 3.

There is no adequate data on intestinal absorption of magnesium in patients with renal failure. The information available is based on calculation of net absorption of magnesium obtained from balance studies. *Clarkson* et al. [33] studied 6 patients with creatinine clearance rates below 30 ml/min and noted that the fraction of magnesium absorbed varied between 0.16 and 0.47. *Kopple and Coburn* [34] found this fraction to range between 0.24 and 0.63. Evaluation of the available data indicates that net magnesium absorption in relation to dietary intake in normal subjects and uremic patients is no different. Thus, it appears that chronic renal failure does not reduce intestinal magnesium absorption and this ion is readily absorbed by these patients independent of the presence of hypermagnesemia, and the body's need for magnesium.

Brannan et al. [35] utilizing jejunal perfusion techniques reported that magnesium absorption is reduced in this segment; they attributed this defect to a deficiency of $1,25(OH)_2D$ [36]. The significance of this finding is not clear. It is possible that a defect in magnesium absorption in uremia is limited to one or two segments of the intestine, while magnesium absorption is probably normal or even increased in other segments; the net result is normal net absorption throughout the entire gut.

References

1   Randall, R.E.; Cohen, M.D.; Spray, C.C.; Rossmeish, E.C.: Hypermagnesemia in renal failure. Etiology and toxic manifestations. Ann. intern. Med. *61*: 73−88 (1964).
2   Wallach, S.; Rizek, J.E.; Dimick, A.; Silver, W.: Magnesium transport in normal and uremic patients. J. clin. Endocr. Metab. *26*: 1069−1080 (1966).

3   Steele, T.H.; Wen, S.F.; Evenson, M.A.; Rieselbach, R.E.: The contribution of chron-
    ically diseased kidney to magnesium homeostasis in man. J. Lab. clin. Med. *71*: 455−463
    (1968).

4   Popovtzer, M.M.; Massry, S.G.; Coburn, J.W.; Kleeman, C.R.: Interrelationship be-
    tween sodium, calcium and magnesium excretion in advanced renal failure. J. Lab. clin.
    Med. *73*: 763−771 (1969).

5   Popovtzer, M.M.; Schainuck, L.I.; Massry, S.G.; Kleeman, C.R.: Divalent ion excre-
    tion in chronic kidney disease. Relation to degree of renal insufficiency. Clin. Sci. *38*:
    297−307 (1970).

6   Coburn, J.W.; Popovtzer, M.M.; Massry, S.G.; Kleeman, C.R.: The physicochemical
    state and renal handling of divalent ions in chronic renal failure. Archs intern. Med.
    124: 302−311 (1969).

7   Gutman, F.D.; Shelp, W.D.; Rieselbach, R.E.: The correlation of fractional excretion
    of sodium and magnesium in the chronically diseased kidney of dog and man. J. Lab.
    clin. Med. *74*: 642−652 (1969).

8   Massry, S.G.; Arieff, A.I.; Coburn, J.W.; Palmieri, G.; Kleeman, C.R.: Divalent ion
    metabolism in patients with acute renal failure. Studies on the mechanism of hypocal-
    cemia. Kidney int. *5*: 437−445 (1974).

9   Smith, W.O.; Hammarstein, J.F.: Serum magnesium in renal diseases. Archs intern.
    Med. *102*: 5−9 (1958).

10 Hanna, S.: Plasma magnesium in health and disease. J. clin. Path. *14*: 410−414 (1961).

11 Walser, M.: Invited discussion. Archs intern. Med. *124*: 292−301 (1969).

12 Ogden, D.A.; Holmes, J.H.: Changes in total and ultrafiltrable plasma calcium and mag-
    nesium during hemodialysis. Trans. Am. Soc. artif. internal Organs *12*: 200−205 (1966).

13 Schmidt, P.; Katzaurek, R.; Zarzgarnik, J.; Hysck, H.: Magnesium metabolism in pa-
    tients on regular dialysis treatment. Clin. Sci. *41*: 131−139 (1971).

14 Blomfield, J.; Wilkinson, C.; Stewart, J.H.; Johnson, J.R.; Wright, R.C.: Control of
    the hypermagnesemia of renal failure by maintenance haemodialysis. Med. J. Austr. *i*:
    854−858 (1970).

15 Massry, S.G.; Coburn, J.W.; Hartenbower, D.L.; Shinaberger, J.H.; Depalma, J.R.;
    Chapman, E.; Kleeman, C.R.: Mineral content of human skin in uremia. Effect of sec-
    ondary hyperparathyroidism and haemodialysis. Proc. Eur. Dial. Transplant Ass. *7*:
    146−150 (1970).

16 Lim, P.; Chin, B.; Dong, S.; Khoo, T.: Intracellular magnesium depletion in chronic
    renal failure. New Engl. J. Med. *280*: 981−984 (1969).

17 Contiguglia, S.R.; Alfrey, A.C.; Miller, N.; Butkus, D.: Total-body magnesium excess
    in chronic renal failure. Lancet *i*: 1300−1302 (1972).

18 Berlyne, G.M.; Ben-Ari, J.; Szwarcberg, J.; Kaneti, J.; Danovitch, G.M.; Kaye, M.:
    Increase in bone magnesium content in renal failure. Nephron *9*: 90−93 (1972).

19 Alfrey, A.C.; Miller, N.: Bone magnesium pools in uremia. J. clin. Invest. *52*:
    3019−3027 (1973).

20 Seelig, M.S.: Requirements of magnesium by normal adult. Summary and analysis of
    published data. Am. J. clin. Nutr. *14*: 242−290 (1964).

21 Dunn, M.J.; Walser, M.: Magnesium depletion in normal man. Metabolism *15*:
    884−895 (1966).

22 Wacker, W.E.C.; Parisi, A.F.: Magnesium metabolism. New Engl. J. Med. *278*:
    658−663, 772−717 (1968).

23 King, R.G.; Stanbury, S.W.: Magnesium metabolism in primary hyperparathyroidism. Clin. Sci. *39*: 218−303 (1970).

24 Avioli, L.V.; Berman, J.: Mg²⁸ kinetics in man. J. appl. Physiol. *21*: 1688−1960 (1966).

25 Graham, L.A.; Coesar, J.J.; Burger, A.S.V.: Gastrointestinal absorption and excretion of Mg²⁸ in man. Metabolism *9*: 646−659 (1960).

26 Fawcett, D.W.; Gens, J.P.: Magnesium poisoning following enema of epsom salt solution. J. Am. med. Ass. *123*: 1028 (1943).

27 Chesley, L.C.; Tepper, I.: Some effects of magnesium loading upon renal excretion of magnesium and certain other electrolytes. J. clin. Invest. *37*: 1362−1372 (1958).

28 Barnes, B.A.; Cope, O.; Harrison, T.: Magnesium conservation in human beings on low magnesium diet. J. clin. Invest. *37*: 430−440 (1958).

29 Alcock, N.; MacIntyre, I.: Interrelation of calcium and magnesium absorption. Clin. Sci. *22*: 185−193 (1962).

30 Heaton, F.W.; Hodgkinson, A.; Rose, G.A.: Observations in the relationship between calcium and magnesium metabolism in man. Clin. Sci. *27*: 31−40 (1964).

31 Clarkson, E.M.; Warren, R.L.; McDonald, S.J.; DeWardener, H.E.: The effect of high intake of calcium on magnesium metabolism in normal subjects and patients with chronic renal failure. Clin. Sci. *32*: 11−18 (1967).

32 Brickman, A.S.; Hartenbower, D.L.; Norman, A.W.; Coburn, J.W.: Action of 1,25(OH)₂ and 1α(OH)-vitamin D₃ on magnesium metabolism in man. Clin. Res. *23*: 315 (1975).

33 Clarkson, E.M.; McDonald, S.J.; DeWardener, H.E.; Warren, R.: Magnesium metabolism in chronic renal failure. Clin. Sci. *28*: 107−115 (1965).

34 Kopple, J.D.; Coburn, J.W.: Metabolic studies of low protein diets in uremia. II. Calcium, phosphorus, and magnesium. Medicine *52*: 597−607 (1973).

35 Brannan, P.G.; Vergne-Marini, P.; Pak, C.Y.C.; Hull, A.R.; Fortran, J.S.: Magnesium absorption in the human small intestine. Results in normal subjects, patients with chronic renal disease and patients with absorptive hypercalciuria. J. clin. Invest. *57*: 1412−1420 (1976).

36 Schmulen, A.C.; Lerman, M.; Pak, C.Y.C.; Zerwekh, J.; Morawaski, S.; Fortran, J.S.; Vergne-Marini, P.: Effect of 1,25-dihydroxyvitamin D therapy of jejunal absorption of magnesium in patients with chronic renal failure. Am. J. Physiol. *238*: 349G-355G (1980).

S.G. Massry, MD, Department of Medicine, Division of Nephrology,
USC School of Medicine, 2025 Zonal Avenue, Los Angeles, CA 90033 (USA)

Contr. Nephrol., vol. 38, pp. 185–194 (Karger, Basel 1984)

Magnesium Load Induced by Ingestion of Magnesium-Containing Antacids

B. Lembcke[a], C. Fuchs[b]

[a]Division of Gastroenterology and Metabolism, Department of Internal Medicine, (Head: Prof. Dr. *W. Creutzfeldt*), [b]Division of Nephrology, Department of Internal Medicine, (Head: Prof. Dr. *F. Scheler*), Göttingen, FRG

Introduction

Antacids are frequently used as a safe, palatable and relatively cheap regimen for the relief of symptoms due to duodenal or gastric ulcer. Concerning the healing of duodenal ulcers, it has been well recognized for years that the neutralizing capacity of the recommended doses is insufficient for an adequate reduction of gastric acidity [1]. *Peterson* et al. [2] recently showed that a large-dose magnesium (Mg) and aluminium (Al) antacid regimen (1,008 mEq of neutralizing capacity) improves the healing of duodenal ulcers. This finding has been reproduced by other authors [3].

However, problems tend to occur where large doses are given for a considerable time. *Peterson* et al. [2] observed substantial diarrhea in two thirds of their patients receiving 210 ml of Mylanta II/day. This side effect can be related to the nonabsorbed Mg moiety acting as an osmotic cahartic due to the formation of unabsorbable Mg salts.

The assumption of prescribing unabsorbed inorganic compounds might be a major factor contributing to the view of safety of antacids, and in general this will hold true. However, some potentially serious side effects may complicate the long-standing administration of sodium bicarbonate ($NaHCO_3$), calcium bicarbonate ($Ca[HCO_3]_2$) or aluminium hydroxide ($Al[OH]_3$) administration (fig. 1).

Most problems of Mg- and Al-containing antacids (if used at a high dosage) result from disturbed bowel habits [2, 4] and from intraluminal antacid-drug interactions [5]. However, both Al and Mg may be absorbed [4, 6, 7]. While Al-induced encephalopathy in patients undergoing dialysis has been recognized as a possible complication of the use of Al-containing

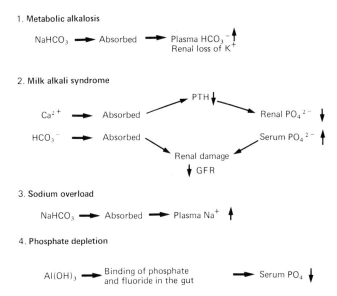

Fig. 1. Side effects of antacids containing sodium bicarbonate, calcium bicarbonate or aluminium hydroxide.

phosphate binders, potential Mg toxicity due to antacid ingestion is less well understood.

The 'Rote Liste' of 1982 comprises 79 chemically defined antacids, 62 of them contain Mg salts or chelates. Few of them, especially those having a good neutralizing capacity, contain a rather high dosage of Mg, e.g. Locid® or Maaloxan®. We have studied the side effects of the latter on serum mineral concentrations and urinary excretion of minerals in healthy subjects. Additionally, alterations of serum Mg, Ca, PO_4 and Al during prophylactic or therapeutic administration of Maaloxan® were studied in a few patients with impaired renal function.

Methods

In the study with healthy volunteers (n = 10), Maaloxan® was administered 7 times daily at a dosage of 30 ml, accounting for a daily intake of 3.5 g Mg and 2.5 g Al (neutralizing capacity: 560 mEq/day). The compound was tested against a placebo; however, due to the significant intestinal side effects of Maaloxan® the double-blind character of the study was biased (increase of bowel movements from 1.4 solid stools/day to 3.6 loose stools/day). During the 4-week antacid (placebo) period, Mg in the serum and the urinary parameters were measured at weekly intervals. Since no significant (p < 0.05) trends were recorded during either period, the mean expression of each parameter during the two periods is given. Among the patients studied, none received the antacid medication for study purposes. As a consequence, different regimen had been applied. All patients were hospitalized on an emergency care or dialysis care unit during the time of study, and all received a high-dosage antacid regimen; details are given in the figures.

Analytical Methods

Plasma and urinary concentrations of Mg, Ca and PO_4 were determined by routine laboratory analysis techniques, in the case of Ca and PO_4 by an automatic analyzing system (Technicon SMAC). Monitoring plasma and urinary Mg concentration in the patients, flameless atomic absorption spectrometry (AAS) was employed. Plasma Al concentrations were measured by flameless AAS using a modification of the technique reported by *Fuchs* et al. [8].

Statistical Evaluation

Statistical evaluation is based on the Wilcoxon matched-pairs, signed-rank test. The values given represent means ± SEM.

Results

Mg Monitoring in Healthy Subjects

In the study with healthy subjects, administration of the antacid led to only a slight increase of serum Mg concentrations (1.71 ± 0.04 vs. 1.60 ± 0.03 mEq/l, p < 0.05). Similar changes occurred with urinary Mg excretion (8.43 ± 0.34 vs. 7.82 ± 0.44 mEq/day, p < 0.05).

Coinciding with the alteration of bowel habits and stool consistency (see 'Introduction'), a reduction of urinary volume from 1,537 ± 162 to 1,173 ± 72 ml/day on taking the antacid was observed (p < 0.01), reflecting the fecal loss of water. Concomitantly urinary pH showed a significant rise from 5.4 ± 0.1 to 6.7 ± 0.2 (p < 0.01), indicating substantial neutralization of gastric acid.

Mg Monitoring in Patients Receiving High-Dosage Antacid Therapy

Case 1. For prevention of cerebral edema following cardiac resuscitation, a 60-year-old patient, R.K. (table I), received dexamethasone therapy. During this phase 200–240 ml Maaloxan®/day was administered by a naso-gastric tube. As far as indicated by serum creatinine concentrations, renal function in this patient was normal. During antacid administration serum Mg increased moderately, thus exceeding the normal range (i.e. 1.4–2.1 mEq/l); however, serum Mg concentrations revealed steady-state conditions.

Table I. Influence of a high dosage Mg and Al antacid regimen (200–240 ml of Maaloxan®/day) on serum Mg, serum Al and urinary Mg excretion in a patient (R.K.) with normal serum creatinine

	Day										
	1	2	3	4	5	6	7	8	9	10	11
Serum Mg, mEq/l	1.99	2.33	2.72	2.20	2.37	2.40	2.22	2.18	2.28	2.33	2.58
Serum Al, µg/l	20	19	19	14	12	13	14	20	16	21	13
Serum creatinine, mg/dl	1.06	0.96	1.64	0.87	0.96	0.92	1.04	1.00	0.96	1.00	1.00
Urine volume ml/day	4,200	4,000	3,290	2,810	4,440	2,720	3,660	3,320	3,980	4,050	3,580
Urinary Mg, mEq/day	13.4	20.08	25.16	30.62	49.28	18.14	25.72	24.33	27.34	28.02	24.66

Increased urinary volume resulted from osmotic and natriuretic diuretics.

Case 2. A rapid and pronounced increase of serum Mg concentration was observed in a 74-year-old patient, K.A. (fig. 2), who was admitted to hospital after having collapsed due to respiratory insufficiency. The underlying cause was purulent pneumonia complicating chronic obstructive lung disease. The patient developed transient renal failure, but did not become anuric. He received 20 ml of Maaloxan® 3–6 times/day beginning on the 4th day after admission, when serum creatinine was 5.2 mg/100 ml. This medication was stopped 6 days later, when the patient was transferred to a normal ward. During this period, maximum serum Mg concentration was 3.99 mEq/l. This concentration was reached within 5 days only. Whether steady-state conditions were achieved in this patient during the 6-day period cannot be definitely decided since there was only one single determination of serum Mg following the peak Mg concentration; however, the Mg profile might support this viewpoint (fig. 2). During the antacid period serum phosphate was significantly reduced while both serum Ca and Al concentrations increased.

Case 3. In another patient (E.B.), extraordinary hypermagnesemia was observed (fig. 3). The patient, E.B., was a 44-year-old female with end-stage renal insufficiency, probably due to both chronic glomerulonephritis and chronic abuse of analgetics, who was on a chronic maintenance hemodialysis program. On Sept. 28, 1981, she took various analgesics and seda-

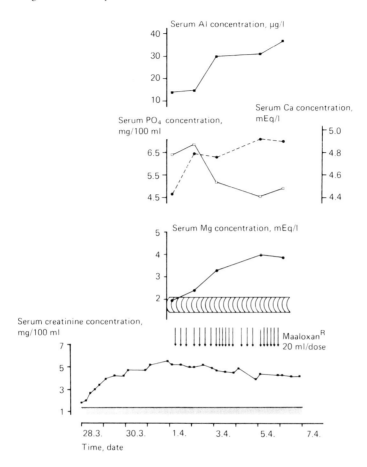

Fig. 2. Effect of a high dosage Mg and Al antacid regimen (60–120 ml Maalocan®/day) on the concentrations of Mg, Ca, Al and PO₄ in the serum of a 74-year-old male patient (K.A.) with impaired renal function. Administation of the antacid was started at peak creatinine concentrations (5.2 mg/100 ml) and stopped 6 days later. The hatched area indicates the normal range of serum Mg concentrations (1.4–2.1 mEq/l). The dotted line refers to serum Ca concentrations.

tives, and then began dialysis at home. 8 h later she was found unarousable with the signs of hypovolemic shock and deep cyanosis. Controlled ventilation and infusion therapy was started at an allocated hospital prior to admission to our clinic few hours later. Hemofiltration was performed and the patient seemed to improve during the next days. Difficulties arose from temperature of unknown origin and bleeding; sepsis was assumed, but no blood culture was found positive. Continuous dopamine administration was required. Finally the patient died

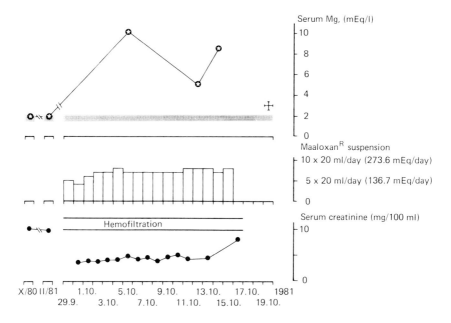

Fig. 3. Alterations of serum Mg concentrations during antacid administration in a 44-year-old female patient (E.B.) with end-stage renal disease. For the patients history see text. Almost normal serum Mg concentrations were registered 8 and 12 months before admission to hospital at the end of September 1981. The patient received 80−160ml Maaloxan®/day (approximately 100−200 mEq of Mg/day). During this period hemofiltration was performed.

from massive cerebral hemorrhage, verified by cranial CT on Oct. 13, 1981. The patient received 20 ml of Maaloxan® 4−8 times/day. After 1 week, the serum Mg concentration was found to be 10.2 mEq/l. Control of this outstanding value revealed a Mg concentration of 5.1 mEq/l (with the medication continued). A second control 2 days later, however, confirmed extreme hypermagnesemia (8.57 mEq/l). Serum Ca at the time of peak Mg concentration was 6.97 mEq/l, and 5.04 and 4.36 mEq/l, respectively, at the two following controls (normal range: 4.48−5.07 mEq/l).

In 6 patients receiving Maaloxan® (4−11 times 20 ml/day), urinary Mg excretion could be monitored for 5−14 days. In all except 1 patient (fig. 4) serum creatinine was normal or only slightly elevated. Serum Mg concentrations in these patients were either normal or, more often, slightly elevated. Maximum serum Mg concentration was 3.16 mEq/l (in the patient with impaired renal function). A close and linear correlation between Mg excretion and urinary volume was observed (fig. 4).

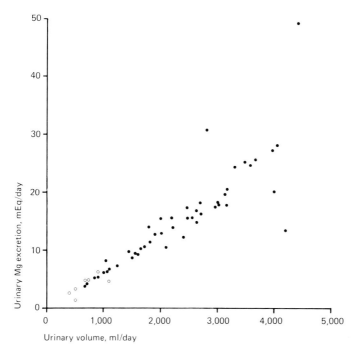

Fig. 4. Correlation of urinary Mg excretion and urinary volume in 6 patients on a high dosage Mg and Al antacid regimen. 5 subjects (●) had normal serum creatinine values. 1 subject (○), with impaired renal function complicating acute pancreatitis, had serum creatinine values of 3.6−7.1 mg/100 ml. The patients were studied for 5, 7, 8, 9, 11 and 14 days, respectively.

Discussion

Normal dietary intake of Mg accounts for 300−350 mg/day [9]. The Mg load induced by Mg-containing antacids may exceed this range manifold, especially if antacids are administered at a dosage which is held necessary for sufficient neutralization of gastric acid [2, 3, 10, 11].

The daily dosage of 210 ml of Maaloxan® administered to healthy subjects during this study contains 3.5 g Mg which equals the Mg load induced by 17.3 g MgSO$_4$. Since Mg may form unabsorbable salts in the gastrointestinal tract, the occurrence of watery diarrhea during the regimen is not surprising. While the serum Mg concentrations in healthy subjects were only slightly affected, urinary volume and pH showed marked alterations which may be of importance for the renal elimination of drugs such as salicylates, quinidine or amphetamines. Further, precipitation of a gray-white sediment could be observed in the urine [4], possibly caused by magnesium-ammonium-phosphate crystals [12]. In our study, urinary Mg excretion showed only a slight increase during the antacid period.

In intensive care units antacids are frequently used for the prevention of acute gastrointestinal hemorrhage. Efficacy, however, has been proven only in a small number of studies with very high dosages of antacids [10, 11]. *Hastings* et al. [10] demonstrated that the incidence of bleeding in severely threatened patients was significantly reduced by hourly gastric instillation of 30 ml Mylanta II (neutralizing capacity 123 mEq/dose), a Mg- and Al-containing antacid. If gastric pH was < 3.5, 60 ml of the antacid was administered. Renal insufficiency was one of the risk factors increasing the incidence of bleeding, thus suggesting antacid administration.

Therefore, we investigated serum Mg concentrations and urinary Mg excretion in a small number of patients who were on a high dosage antacid regimen, few of them having impaired renal function. The data indicate that absorbed Mg leads to an increase of serum Mg concentrations in patients with normal and impaired renal function. With impaired renal function this increase was shown to occur within a few days and serum Mg concentrations tended to be higher (fig. 2). Increased Mg levels due to the administration of antacids, especially in the case of impaired renal function, have been described earlier [6, 7]; however, values around 4 mEq/l (fig. 2) raise the question as to which Mg concentration is toxic. *Randall* et al. [6] reported signs of Mg toxicity at concentrations of 4−5 mEq/l. A remarkable case of oral Mg intoxication was reported in 1975 [13]. This patient showed refractory hypotension sequel to extreme hypermagnesemia (12.5 mEq/l), probably due to abundant absorption from the peritoneal cavity (the patient had perforated duodenal ulcer and the Mg concentration of peritoneal aspirate was 12.2 mEq/l). Patient E.B. (case 3), presented here, had similar serum Mg concentrations (10.2 mEq/l). We must assume that this was due to the ingestion of the Mg- and Al-containing antacid. Since urinary excretion of Mg is related to renal function [6, 9], diminished excretion of the cation is the most likely mechanism of hypermagnesemia in this case. A linear relation of the sodium and Mg clearances has been reported [9]. Among our patients, a linear and close correlation between renal Mg excretion and urinary volume was found in 6 patients (fig. 4), 5 of them having normal serum creatinine values.

Because of potential Mg toxicity, high doses of Mg-containing antacids are contraindicated in patients with impaired renal function. Thus, we are not in agreement with a recent report proposing Mg- and Al-containing antacids for the reduction of serum PO_4 in end-stage renal disease [14]. For the control of gastric acidity, H_2-receptor antagonists are a valuable alternative. However, problems may arise with cimetidine from interactions with other drugs (e.g. β-blockers, theophylline) and accumulation due to decreased glomerular filtration rate, leading to cerebral intoxication [15]. Whether ranitidine has fewer side effects in renal failure still has to be established on a long-term basis.

It is concluded that the administration of Mg-containing antacids in patients with impaired renal function should necessitate repeated measurements of the serum Mg concentrations. In contrast to similar efforts with other drugs like the H_2-receptor antagonists, this 'drug monitoring' (i.e. Mg monitoring) can be more easily performed in clinical practice.

References

1   Holtermüller, K.H.; Bohlen, E.; Castro, M.; Weis, H.J.: Überlegungen zur Therapie mit Antacida. Medsche Klin. *72*: 1229−1241 (1977).

2   Peterson, W.L.; Sturdevant, R.A.L.; Frankl, H.D.; Richardson, C.T.; Isenberg, J.I.; Elashoff, J.D.; Sones, J.Q.; Gross, R.A.; McCallum, R.W.; Fordtran, J.S.: Healing of duodenal ulcer with an antacid regimen. New Engl. J. Med. *297*: 341−345 (1977).

3   Fedeli, G.; Anti, M.; Rapaccini, G.L.; DeVitis, I.; Butti, A.; Civello, I.M.: A controlled study comparing cimetidine treatment to an intensive antacid regimen in the therapy of uncomplicated duodenal ulcer. Dig. Dis. *24*: 758−762 (1979).

4   Lembcke, B.; Fuchs, C.; Hesch, R.D.; Caspary, W.F.: Effects of long-term antacid administration on mineral metabolism; in Halter, Antacids in the eighties, pp. 112−122 (Urban & Schwarzenberg, Munich 1982).

5   Gugler, R.; Musch, E.: Metabolische Wirkungen der Antazida und Interaktionen mit anderen Pharmaka. Z. Gastroent. *21*: suppl., pp. 127−133 (1983).

6   Randall, R.E.; Cohen, M.D.; Spray, C.C.; Rossmeisl, E.C.: Hypermagnesemia in renal failure. Etiology and toxic manifestations. Ann. intern Med. *61*: 73−88 (1964).

7   Bertram, H.P.; Zumkley, H.: Magnesium- und Aluminiumresorption bei Behandlung mit Antazida. Krankenhausarzt *52*: 416−424 (1979).

8   Fuchs, C.; Brasche, M.; Paschen, K.; Nordbeck, H.; Quellhorst, E.: Aluminium-Bestimmung im Serum mit flammenloser Atomabsorption. Clinica chim. Acta *52*: 71−80 (1974).

9   Massry, S.G.: Magnesium metabolism in renal failure; in Cantin, Seelig, Magnesium in health and disease, pp. 439−451 (MTP Press, Lancaster 1980).

10 Hastings, P.R.; Skillman, J.J.; Bushnell, L.S.; Silen, W.: Antacid titration in the prevention of acute gastrointestinal bleeding. New Engl. J. Med. *298*: 1041−1045 (1978).

11 Priebe, H.J.; Skillman, J.J.; Bushnell, L.S.; Long, P.C.; Silen, W.: Antacid versus cimetidine in preventing acute gastorointestinal bleeding. New Engl. J. Med. *302*: 426–430 (1980).

12 Herzog, P.; Schmitt, K.F.; Grendahl, T.; van der Linden, J.; Holtermüller, K.H.: Evaluation of serum and urine electrolyte changes during therapy with a magnesium-aluminium-containing antacid: results of a prospective study: in Halter, Antacids in the eighties, pp. 123–135 (Urban & Schwarzenberg, Munich 1982).

13 Mordes, J.P.; Swartz, R.; Arky, R.A.: Extreme hypermagnesemia as a cause of refractory hypotension. Ann. intern Med. *83*: 657–658 (1975).

14 Guillot, A.P.; Hood, V.L.; Runge, C.F.; Gennari, F.J.: The use of magnesium-containing phosphate binders in patients with end-stage renal disease on maintenance hemodialysis. Nephron *30*: 114–117 (1982).

15 Reinmann, I.; Klotz, U.: Klinisch bedeutsame Interaktionen von Cimetidin. Inn. Med. *10*: 31–40 (1983).

Dr. med. Bernhard Lembcke, Medizinische Klinik und Poliklinik der Universität Göttingen, Robert-Koch-Strasse 40, D-3400 Göttingen (FRG)

Contr. Nephrol., vol. 38, pp. 195–202 (Karger, Basel 1984)

Does Magnesium Excess Play a Role in Renal Osteodystrophy?

T. Drüeke

Département de Néphrologie, Hôpital Necker, Paris, France

Disturbed Mg Metabolism in Uremia

The metabolism of magnesium is considerably altered in chronic renal failure. An increase in plasma Mg concentration is common in patients with acute [1] and chronic renal failure on conservative treatment [2–5]. The percentage of serum Mg not bound to protein was found to be $76 \pm 8\%$ in uremic patients, a value no different from $75 \pm 9\%$ observed in normal persons [4]. Mg concentrations were increased in sweat [6] and in parotid saliva [7] from chronic renal failure patients. Tissue Mg concentrations have been reported to be normal [8–10], increased [11–15], or diminished [16]. The reasons for these divergent results are not clear. The studies of *Lim* et al. [16] were carried out in Hong Kong, where dietary Mg may have been quite low [17]. It is also possible that Mg concentrations in different tissues are not all equally representative of total body Mg stores. The muscle Mg content could be quite insensitive to changes in the body stores, while a labile skeletal pool may reflect more closely an increase or decrease in Mg [18, 19].

Varying degrees of chronic renal failure, different types of underlying nephropathy, more or less pronounced concomitant disturbances of phosphate and calcium metabolism as well as the amount of dietary Mg intake and absorption may all contribute to the generally disturbed metabolism of magnesium in patients with chronic renal failure.

Intestinal Mg absorption in uremia has been found to be normal or decreased [5, 20–22]. It must be noted that marked differences existed between individual patients when undergoing metabolic balance studies [5, 20–22]. Net absorption of Mg was greater during a higher Mg intake [22].

When increasing dietary Ca intake moderately no change in Mg absorption was noted in patients with chronic renal failure [5, 22]. However, the oral administration of large quantities of Ca led to a decrease in serum Mg [23], possibly owing to reduced intestinal Mg absorption. Ingestion of laxatives or antacids which contain Mg can substantially augment the total intake of Mg [3, 24, 25]. Vitamin D and its active metabolites or derivatives had either no effect [26] or stimulated [27, 28] intestinal absorption of Mg in uremic animals and patients. Urinary Mg excretion was reported to be low [20, 22] or normal [5] in uremic patients.

In uremic patients treated with regular dialysis, the Mg balance is affected not only by the dietary intake and urinary excretion but also by the dialysate concentration of Mg [4, 8, 29−33]. The movement of Mg across the dialysis membrane depends upon its diffusible electrochemical gradient between the blood and the dialysate [29]. Thus, high Mg losses into the dialysis fluid were observed in hemodialyzed patients when the dialysate Mg was as low as 0.27 mg/100 ml [30]. An increase in plasma Mg concentration has been found in such patients when a dialysis fluid was utilized containing 1.8 mg/100 ml of Mg, a decrease when the dialysis fluid contained only 0.6 mg/100 ml of Mg [4]. Similarly, elevated serum Mg levels and a positive Mg balance were reported in uremic patients treated by continuous ambulatory peritoneal dialysis with a relatively high dialysate Mg concentration [32, 33]. In hemodialysis patients dialyzed against a high dialysate Mg concentration, an increased content of Mg in the skin has also been demonstrated [11].

The observations summarized above suggest that chronically uremic patients are prone to develop hypermagnesemia. They may absorb normal amounts of Mg inspite of a reduced renal capacity for excreting the absorbed Mg. Hemodialysis and peritoneal dialysis may further add Mg to the uremic organism if dialysate Mg concentrations are sufficiently high. Taken together these changes in Mg metabolism can lead to Mg excess in at least some of the patients with chronic renal failure.

Potential Role of Mg in Uremic Bone Disease

The calcification process of bone is still poorly understood [31]. Amongst possible inhibitors of crystallization, such as pyrophosphate, diphosphonates, citrate, and proteoglycans, the Mg ion appears also to be a serious candidate. Mg is known to stabilize amorphous calcium phosphate and thereby to inhibit apatite crystal formation in vitro [34, 35]. Mg has been found to be surface-located in relation to the crystal lattice [36], a finding which could be important to the interpretation of its possible inhibitory function. It has been hypothesized that Mg could combine with pyrophosphate (P_2O_7) to form MgP_2O_7. The latter has been shown to be particularly resistant to hydrolysis by the enzyme, pyrophosphatase, at least in brain tissue [37]. Thus, permanently high concentrations of MgP_2O_7 could inhibit amorphous calcium phosphate in bone as well as soft tissue deposits to be transformed into apatite [38]. In this context it is also of note that Mg has been reported to potentiate metastatic calcifications in vitamin D-treated rats [39].

In addition to its possible direct effect on the calcification process at bone level, Mg could also exert an indirect effect on bone turnover by influencing parathyroid hormone secretion. Since the Mg ion is an activator for a large number of enzymes including alkaline phosphatase and Ca-Mg-ATPase in many tissues, the existence of a high affinity Ca-Mg-ATPase in parathyroid tissue [40] was not unexpected. In a recent in vitro study, Mg has been shown to stimulate parathyroid hormone secretion [41]. This effect was attributed to a possible activation by Mg of parathyroid adenylate cyclase via endogenous guanine nucleotides. Conversely, the stimulation of hormonal secretion could also have been due to a competition of Mg with Ca for binding to a distinct regulatory site on adenylate cyclase [41]. However, in previous in vitro experiments elevated extracellular Mg concentrations were found to suppress parathyroid hormone secretion [42–44]. Varying experimental conditions including different animal species used for tissue sampling, different states of previous Mg load, and different assay procedures are probably at the cause of such divergent results. In the human situation in the absence of renal failure, the response of the parathyroid glands to acute i.v. Mg infusions was also different depending on the patients' underlying disease. In hyperparathyroid patients, either no change or an inhibition of parathyroid hormone secretion was observed, whereas in patients with chronic Mg deficiency, the acute elevation in serum Mg concentration led to an immediate rise in the hormone's serum concentration [45]. The chronic Mg-deficient state is associated with a decrease in plasma parathyroid hormone concentration [45]. The effect of a chronic Mg overload in vivo in the presence of normal renal function does not seem to have been examined [17]. Thus, Mg could influence bone metabolism either by directly affecting the crystallization process or indirectly by modifying parathyroid hormone secretion.

During chronic renal failure an increase in bone Mg content has been observed in experimental animal studies [46] as well as in the majority of studies performed in patients [10, 12, 15, 47−49]. The increase in bone Mg was associated with a concomitant decrease in the carbonate content [47, 48] but an increase in the phosphate content [48] of bone mineral. *Burnell* et al. [47] and *Pellegrino* et al. [48] made the hypothesis that such a Mg excess could contribute to the often observed maturational defect in uremic bone. Indeed, Mg changes were inversely related to Ca changes in bone mineral, and a correlation existed between bone mineral Mg and osteoid [48]. *Alfrey and Solomons* [15] attributed to the Mg salt of pyrophosphate, MgP_2O_7, a possible inhibitory role in the calcification process of uremic bone, since both Mg and pyrophosphate contents were found increased in the bones of uremic patients examined in their study. Mg-pyrophosphate seems particularly resistant to hydrolysis by pyrophosphatase [37]. Excess Mg could also directly inhibit the activity of bone alkaline phosphatase and thereby lead to an increase in bone pyrophosphate content and thus interfere with the normal crystallization process [17, 47].

Several studies of exogenous Mg supplementation have been performed in uremic animals and patients in order to explore the possibility of a beneficial effect on parathyroid function and thus the skeleton. *Kaye* [46] administered a high Mg intake to chronically uremic rats during 4 weeks. He observed not a decrease, but an increase in parathyroid gland weight and in bone resorption. *Pletka* et al. [31] and *Ritz* et al. [50] dialyzed uremic patients against a high dialysis fluid Mg concentration (2.5 mEq/l) in order to obtain a positive Mg balance. The former observed a decrease in serum immunoreactive parathyroid hormone, calcium, and phosphorus concentration during a 2-month treatment and suggested a possibly beneficial effect on bone resorption. The latter, however, failed to find a change of the circulating parathyroid hormone level. They attributed this to the concomitant relatively high dialysate Ca concentration (3.5 mEq/l) used for their patients, which is known to be associated with a better control of hyperparathyroidism at the bone level [51−53]. In neither of the two clinical studies with high dialysate Mg concentrations were bone analyses performed in order to substantiate the conclusions based on biochemical determinations. *Coburn* et al. [4] found no correlation between diffusible serum Mg and serum inorganic phosphorus or ionized Ca.

A warning against the creation of a positive Mg balance by high exogenous Mg intake has very recently been formulated on the basis of the observation that the administration of Mg-containing phosphate binders to dialysis patients was associated with a high incidence of fracturing osteomalacia [25]. The latter disappeared after the replacement of these binders by Mg-free phosphate binders. This seemed to exclude a primary role of aluminium.

Taken together, the above summarized observations lead us to conclude, in full agreement with *David* [17], that the iatrogenic induction of a positive Mg balance in uremic patients via the oral or the dialytic route is unphysiological and might be hazardous. Even if a beneficial effect could be obtained, at least in some cases, in terms of a better control of hyperparathyroidism, an interference of excess Mg with the mineralization process of bone may possibly exist. This could lead to a decrease of hydroxyapatite formation in bone and in addition to an increase in visceral calcification, even though nonvisceral (hydroxyapatite-composed) extraskeletal calcification could be theoretically diminished. Therefore, the presently available evidence suggests that Mg excess should be avoided in patients with chronic renal failure.

References

1   Hamburger, J.: Electrolyte disturbance in acute uremia. Clin. Chem. *3*: 332–343 (1975).

2   Robinson, R.R.; Murdaugh, H.V., Jr.; Peschel, E.: Renal factors responsible for the hypermagnesemia of renal disease. J. Lab. clin. Med. *53*: 572–576 (1959).

3   Randall, R.E. , Jr.; Cohen, M.D.; Spray, C.C.; Rossmeisl, E.C.: Hypermagnesemia in renal failure. Etiology and toxic manifestations. Ann. intern. Med. *61*: 73–88 (1964).

4   Coburn, J.W.; Popovtzer, M.M.; Massry, S.G.; Kleeman, C.R.: The physicochemical state and renal handling of divalent ions in chronic renal failure. Archs. intern. Med. *124*: 302–311 (1969).

5   Kopple, J.D.; Coburn, J.W.: Metabolic studies of low protein diets in uremia. II. Calcium, phosphorus and magnesium. Medicine, Baltimore *52*: 597–607 (1973).

6   Prompt, C.A.; Quinton, P.M.; Kleeman, C.R.: High concentrations of sweat calcium, magnesium and phosphate in chronic renal failure. Nephron *20*: 4–9 (1978).

7   Earlbaum, A.M.; Quinton, P.M.: Elevated divalent ion concentrations in parotid saliva from chronic renal failure patients. Nephron *28*: 58–61 (1981).

8   Catto, G.R.D.; Reid, I.W.; MacLeod, M.: The effect of low magnesium dialysate on plasma, ultrafiltrable, erythrocyte and bone magnesium concentrations from patients on maintenance hemodialysis. Nephron *13*: 372–381 (1974).

9   Wallach, S.; Rizek, J.E.; Dimich, A.; Prasad, N.; Siler, W.: Magnesium transport in normal and uremic patients. J. clin. Endocr. Metab. *26*: 1069–1080 (1966).

10 Lim, P.; Jacob, E.: Magnesium status in chronic uremic patients. Nephron *9*: 300–307 (1972).

11 Massry, S.G.; Coburn, J.W.; Hartenbower, D.L.; Shinaberger, J.H.; DePalma, J.R.; Chapman, E.; Kleeman, C.R.: Mineral content of human skin in uremia. Effect of sec-

ondary hyperparathyroidism and hemodialysis. Proc. Eur. Dial. Transplant Ass. 7: 146–150 (1970).

12   Contiguglia, S.R.; Alfrey, A.C.; Miller, N.; Butkus, D.: Total body mangesium excess in chronic renal failure. Lancet i: 1300–1302 (1972).

13   Berlyne, G.M.; Ben-Air, J.; Szwarcberg, J.; Kaneti, J.; Danovitch, G.M.; Kaye, M.: Increase in bone magnesium content in chronic renal failure in man. Nephron 9: 90–93 (1972).

14   Alfrey, A.C.; Miller, N.L.: Bone magnesium pools in uremia. J. clin. Invest. 52: 3019–3027 (1973).

15   Alfrey, A.C.; Solomons, C.C.: Bone pyrophosphate in uremia and its association with extraosseous calcification. J. clin. Invest. 57: 700–705 (1976).

16   Lim, P.; Dong, S.; Khoo, D.T.: Intracellular magnesium depletion in chronic renal failure. New Engl. J. Med. 280: 981–984 (1969).

17   David, S.D.: Mineral and bone homeostasis in renal failure: pathophysiology and management; in David, Calcium metabolism in renal failure and nephrolithiasis, pp. 1–76 (Wiley, New York 1977).

18   Smith, R.H.: Calcium and magnesium metabolism in calves. Biochem. J. 71: 609–615 (1959).

19   Alfrey, A.C.; Miller, N.L.; Butkus, D.: Evaluation of body magnesium stores. J. Lab. clin. Med. 84: 153–162 (1974).

20   Clarkson, E.M.; McDonald, S.J.; Wardener, H.E. de; Warren, R: Magnesium metabolism in chronic renal failure. Clin. Sci. 28: 107–115 (1965).

21   Brannan, P.G.; Vergne-Marini, P.; Pak, C.Y.C.; Hull, A.R.; Fordtran, J.S.: Magnesium absorption in the human small intestine. J. clin. Invest. 57: 1412–1418 (1976).

22   Spencer, H.; Lesniak, M.; Gatza, C.A.; Osis, D.; Lender, M.: Magnesium absorption and metabolism in patients with chronic renal failure and in patients with normal renal function. Gastroenterology 79: 26–34 (1980).

23   Popovtzer, M.M.; Robinette, J.B.: Effect of oral calcium carbonate on urinary excretion of Ca, Na and Mg in advanced renal disease. Proc. Soc. exp. Biol. Med. 145: 222–226 (1974).

24   Guillot, A.P.; Hood, V.L.; Runge, C.F.; Gennari, F.J.: The use of magnesium-containing phosphate binders in patients with end-stage renal disease on maintenance hemodialysis. Nephron 30: 114–117 (1982).

25   Brunner, F.P.; Thiel, G.: Re: The use of magnesium-containing phosphate binders in patients with end-stage renal disease on maintenance hemodialysis (letter). Nephron 32: 226 (1982).

26   Kanis, J.A.; Smith, R.; Walton, R.J.; Barlett, M.: Effect of 1-alpha-hydroxycholecalciferol on magnesium metabolism in chronic renal failure. Br. med. J. i: 211 (1977).

27   Meintzer, R.B.; Steenbock, H.: Vitamin D and magnesium absorption. J. Nutr. 56: 285–294 (1955).

28   Schmulen, A.C.; Lerman, M.; Pak, Y.C.Y.; Zerwek, J.; Morawski, S.; Fordtran, J.S.; Vergne-Marini, P.: Effect of $1,25(OH)_2$-D_3 on jejunal absorption of magnesium in patients with chronic renal disease. Am. J. Physiol. 238: 349–352 (1980).

29   Ogden, D.A.; Holmes, J.H.: Changes in total and ultrafilterable plasma calcium and magnesium during hemodialysis. Trans. Am. Soc. artif, internal Organs 12: 200–204 (1966).

30 Schmidt, P.; Kotzaurek, R.; Zazgornik, J.; Hysek, H.: Magnesium metabolism in patients on regular dialysis treatment. Clin. Sci. *41*: 131−139 (1971).

31 Pletka, P.; Bernstein, D.S.; Hampers, C.L.; Merrill, J.P.; Sherwood, L.M.: Relationship between magnesium and secondary hyperparathyroidism during long-term hemodialysis. Metabolism *23*: 619−630 (1974).

32 Delmez, J.A.; Slatopolsky, E.; Martin, K.J.; Gearing, B.N.; Harter, H.R.: Minerals, vitamin D, and parathyroid hormone in continuous ambulatory peritoneal dialysis. Kidney int. *21*: 862−867 (1982).

33 Blumenkrantz, M.J.; Kopple, J.D.; Moran, J.K.; Coburn, J.W.: Metabolic balance studies and dietary protein requirements in patients undergoing continuous ambulatory peritoneal dialysis. Kidney int. *21*: 849−861 (1982).

34 Bachra, B.N.; Trantz, O.R.; Simon, S.L.: Precipitation of calcium carbonates and phosphates. III. The effect of magnesium and fluoride ions on the spontaneous precipitation of calcium carbonates and phosphates. Archs. oral. Biol. *10*: 731−738 (1965).

35 Fleisch, H.: Mechanisms of calcification; in Massry, Ritz, Phosphate and minerals in health and disease, Adv. exp. Med. Biol., vol. 128, pp. 563−577 (Plenum Press, New York 1980).

36 Neuman, W.F.; Mulryan, B.J.: Synthetic hydroxyapatite crystals. IV. Magnesium incorporation. Calcif. Tissue Res. *7*: 133−138 (1971).

37 Cathala, G.; Brunel, C.: L'activité pyrophosphatasique de la phosphatase alcaline du cerveau. Biochim. biophys. Acta *315*: 73−82 (1973).

38 Alfrey, A.C.; Solomons, C.C.; Ciricillo, J.; Miller, N.L.: Extraosseous calcification. Evidence for abnormal pyrophosphate metabolism in uremia. J. clin. Invest. *57*: 692−699 (1976).

39 Whittier, F.C.; Freeman, R.M.: Potentiation of metastatic calcification in vitamin D-treated rats by magnesium. Am. J. Physiol. *220*: 209−212 (1971).

40 Dawson-Hughes, B.; Brown, E.M.: $(Ca^{++}-Mg^{++})$ATPase activity in bovine parathyroid cells. Clin. Res. *29*: 681 A (1981).

41 Mahaffee, D.D.; Cooper, C.W.; Ramp, W.K.; Ontjes, D.A.: Magnesium promotes both parathyroid hormone secretion and adenosine 3′,5′-monophosphate production in rat parathyroid tissues and reverses the inhibitory effects of calcium on adenylate cyclase. Endocrinology *110*: 487−495 (1982).

42 Targovnik, J.H.; Rodman, J.S.; Sherwood, L.M.: Regulation of parathyroid hormone secretion in vitro: quantitative aspects of calcium and magnesium ion control. Endocrinology *88*: 1477−1482 (1971).

43 Habener, J.F.; Potts, J.T., Jr.: Relative effectiveness of magnesium and calcium on the secretion and biosynthesis of parathyroid hormone in vitro. Endocrinology *98*: 197−202 (1976).

44 Sherwood, L.M.; Hanley, D.A.; Takatsuki, K.; Birnbaumer, M.E.; Schneider, A.B.; Wells, S.A., Jr.: Regulation of parathyroid hormone secretion; in Copp, Talmage, Endocrinology of Calcium Metabolism, pp. 301−307 (Excerpta Medica, Amsterdam 1978).

45 Rude, R.K.; Oldham, S.B.; Sharp, C.F.; Singer, FR: Parathyroid hormone secretion in magnesium deficiency. J. clin. Endocr. Metab. *47*: 800−806 (1978).

46 Kaye, M.: Magnesium metabolism in the rat with chronic renal failure. J. Lab. clin. Med. *84*: 536−545 (1974).

47 Burnell, J.M.; Teubner, E.; Wergedal, J.E.; Sherrard, D.J.: Bone crystal maturation in renal osteodystrophy in humans J. clin. Invest. *53*: 52−58 (1974).

48   Pellegrino, E.D.; Biltz, R.M.; Letteri, J.M.: Interrelationships of carbonate, phos-
     phate, monohydrogen phosphate, calcium, magnesium, and sodium in uraemic bone:
     comparison of dialysed and non-dialysed patients. Clin. Sci. mol. Med. *53*: 307–316
     (1977).
49   Sieberth, H.G.; Von Baeyer, H.; Ritz, E.: Bone mineral content and bone mass in
     uremic and hemodialyzed patients (Abstract). 22nd Annu. Meet. Am. Soc. Artif. In-
     tern. Organs, San Francisco 1976, p. 74.
50   Ritz, E.; Lenhard, V.; Bommer, J.; Hackeng, W.: The effect of dialysate magnesium
     concentration on serum PTH levels in patients on maintenance hemodialysis. Klin.
     Wschr. *52*: 51–53 (1974).
51   Ritz, E.; Malluche, H.; Bommer, J.; Mehls, O.; Krempien, B.: Metabolic bone disease
     in patients on maintenance hemodialysis. Nephron *12*: 393–404 (1974).
52   Fournier, A.E.; Johnson, W.J.; Traves, D.R.; Beabout, J.W.; Arnaud, C.D.;
     Goldsmith, R.S.: Etiology of hyperparathyroidism and bone disease during chronic
     hemodialysis. I. Association of bone disease with potentially etiologic factors. J. clin.
     Invest. *50*: 592–598 (1971).
53   Drüeke, T.; Bordier, P.J.; Man, N.K.; Jungers, P.; Marie, P.: Effects of high dialysate
     calcium concentration on bone remodelling, serum biochemistry, and parathyroid hor-
     mone in patients with renal osteodystrophy. Kidney int. *11*: 267–274 (1977).

Dr. T. Drüeke, Prof. associé, Département de Néphrologie, Hôpital Necker,
161, rue de Sèvres, F-75743 Paris Cédex 15 (France)

Contr. Nephrol., vol. 38, pp. 203–204 (Karger, Basel 1984)

Discussion: Magnesium Metabolism

In the discussion, *Massry* firstly referred to the effects of vitamin D and its metabolites on renal handling of various electrolytes (magnesium, calcium and inorganic phosphate). He especially stressed the different actions of acute and chronic vitamin D administration. In the acute experiment, the U/P ratio of phosphate and − according to some investigators − the plasma concentration of ADH and calcitonin as modifying factors have to be taken into consideration. However, direct actions of vitamin D or its metabolites seem probable.

During chronic administration of vitamin D, the increased filtered load of calcium and the altered U/P ratio of phosphate create changes in tubular electrolyte handling, interfering with the vitamin D action.

A second point of discussion concerned the high fractional Mg excretion in renal insufficiency in spite of the elevated plasma concentration of PTH. In order to explain this phenomenon *Massry* underscored the potential modifying role of the natriuretic hormone, which inhibits the reabsorption of sodium, calcium, phosphate and magnesium in the proximal tubule and thereby enhances the fluid delivery to the distal renal tubule. In this part of the nephron, PTH normally stimulates magnesium reabsorption, which in renal insufficiency is overcome by the increased fluid delivery.

Ritz asks whether high magnesium levels in the serum inhibit the synthesis of PTH or suppress its exocytosis. In this connection he pointed out the in vitro experiments performed by *Raisz*, who demonstrated that magnesium only suppressed the release of PTH into the incubation medium but did not alter the incorporation of labelled leucine, meaning an unchanged PTH synthesis.

Heidland recalled earlier investigations indicating an enhanced tubular reabsorption of magnesium after administration of the potassium-sparing diuretics triamteren and amiloride. Analogous to the acute effects of PTH these diuretics raise the urinary pH, which possibly has some importance for enhanced tubular reabsorption of magnesium.

In the context of potassium-sparing diuretics, *Massry* pointed out that in all hypomagnesic states there is a concomitant hypopotassemia: however, on the contrary, hypopotassemia is not always associated with hypomagnesemia. Finally, he underlined the magnesium-, calcium- and potassium-wasting effects of the various aminoglycoside antibiotics.

One participant mentioned the potential role of elevated serum magnesium level for vascular calcification (deposition of amorphous calcium, magnesium and phosphate complexes) in hemodialysis patients.

In the last discussion point, *Massry* mentioned the enhanced calcium deposition in various organs in experimental uremia of dogs (2−3 years duration). The disturbance could be observed even in the presence of normal serum phosphate. PTX in these animals decreased the calcium accumulation in the tissues, but did not normalise the calcium content.

In patients with chronic renal failure, *Massry* observed tremendous calcification, particularly in the lung tissue, using the technetium scanning technique.

Discussion to the Paper of Lembcke: First the patellar reflex is pointed as a simple clinical criterium, which as long it is positive excludes a dangerous hypermagnesemia. The further discussion reminds one of the dependence of magnesium toxicity on the blood calcium concentration and makes clear (*Ritz, Massry*) that hypermagnesemia cannot be caused by ingestion of antacids alone but also by hypercatabolic or febrile states. In these situations as well as in oliguria magnesium-containing antacids should not be used. Therefore, and because of their interactions with other drugs and their effects on water and electrolytes in the intestines such antacids no longer should be given on a routine basis to severely ill patients in intensive care units to prevent gastrointestinal bleeding.

Discussion to the Paper of Drüeke: Some questions concerning the usefulness of a magnesium-free dialysate are answered by *Drüeke*: He recommends it only for patients with a regular intake of magnesium-containing antacids. Otherwise, concentrations between 0.8 and 1.2 mval/l seem to be appropriate. One speaker refers to the observation that one organ, the myocardium, is depleted of magnesium in chronic renal insufficiency. The question (*Eschbach*) as to which serum concentration of magnesium would represent a borderline of toxicity cannot be answered exactly.

Prof. *A. Heidland, Würzburg*
Prof. *E. Wetzels, Rosenheim*

Subject Index